Weighing the Evidence

How is birthweight determined?

Nick Spencer

Professor of Child Health
School of Health and Social Studies
School of Postgraduate Medical Education
University of Warwick

T0133919

Radcliffe Medical Press

Radcliffe Medical Press Ltd
18 Marcham Road
Abingdon
Oxon OX14 1AA
United Kingdom

www.radcliffe-oxford.com
The Radcliffe Medical Press electronic catalogue and online ordering facility.
Direct sales to anywhere in the world.

© 2003 Nick Spencer

All rights reserved. No part of this publication may be reproduced, stored in a retrieval system
or transmitted, in any form or by any means, electronic, mechanical, photocopying,
recording or otherwise without the prior permission of the copyright owner.

British Library Cataloguing in Publication Data

A catalogue record for this book is available from the British Library.

ISBN 1 85775 594 4

Typeset by Advance Typesetting Ltd, Oxfordshire
Printed and bound by TJ International Ltd, Padstow, Cornwall

Contents

Acknowledgements

My first acknowledgement is to an academic and researcher whom I have not met but whose influence is evident throughout the book. Anyone interested in the determinants of birthweight and gestational duration very quickly becomes familiar with the work of Dr Michael Kramer. His contribution to this field of study is truly Olympian. His work provides the framework for much of this book, especially Chapters 4 and 5, and I hope he will forgive me for using his material as a constant reference point throughout the book.

I owe an immense debt to Professor John Emery who died recently in a tragic accident. John, although a paediatric pathologist, understood the relationship between the biological and the social and persuaded me, along with many other young paediatricians fortunate enough to come under his influence, to look beyond the narrow confines of acute paediatrics and begin to address the social influences on biological phenomena. Professor Sir David Hull must also take some of the credit for encouraging my nascent interest in academic community child health. In the 1970s, academic community child health barely existed but David's foresight and encouragement helped me to gain the confidence to venture into this new area.

Thanks to John Emery, I became a member of the European Society of Social Paediatrics (ESSOP) in the late 1970s and have been privileged to work with, and count among my friends, many of the leading thinkers in social paediatrics in Europe including Lennart Kohler, Michel Manciaux, Bengt Lindstrom and Claus Sundelin. ESSOP provides an international forum for those interested in the social influences on child health and my ideas have been enriched by academic contact with Australian and American colleagues such as Frank Oberklaid, Garth Alperstein, Victor Nossar, Shanti Raman, Bob Chamberlain and Bob Greenberg.

My long and fruitful collaboration and friendship with Professor Stuart Logan has profoundly influenced my understanding of the causal mechanisms by which health is determined. Over the course of our prolonged and often frustrating battle to insist, against the prevailing orthodoxy, on the importance of social influences on child health, Stuart's command of epidemiology has provided me with a firm scientific base on which to develop my ideas. Dr Aidan Macfarlane, one of the first UK community consultant paediatricians, has been a constant source of encouragement in my academic development.

I would not have been able to complete this book without the help of Dianne Forster and Wendy Higman, research assistants in the School of Postgraduate Medical Education, who undertook extensive literature searches for projects related to birthweight and preterm birth. The literature reviewed in this book was mainly obtained with their help. My colleagues in the School of Health and Social Studies, notably Clare Blackburn and Chris Coe, have provided me with invaluable support and encouragement. My thanks also go to the University of Warwick for awarding me generous study leave to write this book and to my paediatric colleagues in Coventry who have shouldered extra work in order to free me to write.

Finally, I would like to thank my wife, Anthea, for her constant encouragement and enthusiasm for my academic work and my children, Justin, Gareth and Tim, my grandchildren, Charlotte and Luis, and my step-children, Phoebe and Tom, for allowing me time to complete this book.

Introduction

Birthweight marks both a beginning and an end, an alpha and an omega. It is a pivotal measure in the life course reflecting the intergenerational transmission of risk and protective influences as well as contributing to the future shape of the life course through childhood into adulthood. Although frequently characterised as a biological variable, birthweight is an example of the complex interplay between biological, social and psychological factors that is manifest at population level as social gradients, ethnic differences and differences in birthweight distributions between countries.

Birthweight is not the only important measure at birth; length and head circumference are important markers of pregnancy outcome and also contribute to the future life course. However, birthweight is the most commonly and accurately measured, and most widely studied, birth measure. In countries in which infants are routinely weighed and measured at birth, weight is the measure given greatest attention by parents to the extent that it is accurately recalled by mothers as many as 20 years after the birth. The special place of birthweight in research and lay perceptions justifies making it the focus of this book.

Birthweight along with gestational age have long been recognised as the main determinant of neonatal and infant mortality and morbidity. In response to the greatly increased risk of adverse neonatal outcomes among infants weighing less than 2500g and those born early, research on the determinants of birthweight and gestational age has focused on the lower extremes of the distribution. While this research has identified important risk factors, examination across the whole birthweight range including population means and distributions throws additional light on how birthweight is determined. For this reason, this book is concerned with the determinants of birthweight rather than low birthweight or preterm birth and attempts to combine the large volume of evidence related to risk factors for low birthweight and preterm birth with the much smaller evidence base related to the whole birthweight range.

The study of the relationship between birthweight and subsequent cardiovascular mortality among men in adult life[1] provided the impetus for the development of life course epidemiology.[2] Birthweight is not only linked to neonatal and infant survival and a range of childhood health outcomes but is now known to be associated with cognitive function and educational attainment in later childhood and into adulthood, adult height and a range of adult health outcomes (*see* Chapter 2). Thus, birthweight has a long reach across the full extent of the life course. As a result, birthweight has taken on a new importance for public health.

Given the extensive literature on the determinants and consequences of birthweight, it is reasonable to question the need for a book such as this. Arising from my interest in the social determinants of child health, I have developed a growing interest in the social gradient in birthweight, why it occurs and what can be done to attenuate it. Study of the social gradient has led me to consider the mechanisms by which social and socially-related factors influence biological processes to produce smaller infants. I have also been struck by the fact that, despite the upsurge in interest in birthweight as a determinant of events later in the life course, few studies have used life course epidemiology to explore the determinants of birthweight itself. This book aims to construct theoretical models of birthweight determination incorporating social, biological and psychological factors acting across generations and over time that can be tested in empirical research. A further aim is to refocus the debate on prevention of low birthweight and preterm birth. Preventive strategies have been disappointing (*see* Chapter 6). This is likely to be related to the use of interventions aiming to modify single proximal risk factors. The biological processes initiated by the biopsychosocial pathways may well be too far advanced for interventions late in the index pregnancy to have anything other than a marginal effect. Elucidation of the pathways should inform new approaches to prevention.

The first part of the book considers the evidence for the effect that birthweight exerts on the life course. The effects of birthweight in childhood are considered in the first chapter, followed by the effects into adult life. The final chapter of this part examines the public health importance of birthweight along with trends and international comparisons.

Part 2 details the evidence related to social, psychological and biological determinants of birthweight. The final chapter of this part draws this evidence together to model biopsychosocial pathways to birthweight based on the principles of life course epidemiology taking account of distal as well as proximal factors and intergenerational effects.

Part 3 considers the possible reasons for the poor performance of interventions aimed at preventing low birthweight and preterm birth before moving on to consider new preventive approaches based on the biopsychosocial pathways modelled in Part 2 and an extended model including societal level influences on individual level variables. The penultimate chapter explores the health and social policy implications of the models and future research directions. The final chapter briefly summarises the main themes of the book.

References

1 Barker DJ (ed) (1992) *Fetal and Infant Origins of Adult Disease*. BMJ Publications, London.

2 Kuh D and Ben-Shlomo Y (eds) (1997) *A Life Course Approach to Chronic Disease Epidemiology*. Oxford University Press, Oxford.

PART I

The importance of birthweight

CHAPTER I

Birthweight and health in childhood

The objective of the first part of this book is to establish birthweight as a measure of public health importance with major health and social policy implications. This chapter summarises the impact of birthweight on health in childhood. Birthweight as a key determinant of mortality in infancy and childhood is considered, followed by the relationship of birthweight to a range of neurodevelopmental, sensory and other health outcomes in childhood. Next, evidence for the impact of birthweight on cognitive function, school readiness and educational attainment is summarised. Finally factors related to socio-economic status and ethnicity that may act to modify birthweight effects are considered.

As discussed in the Introduction, the evidence for the effects of birthweight on child health outcomes is dominated by studies of low birthweight and preterm infants. In calling on this evidence it is important to stress that the consequences of being born early (less than 37 weeks' gestation) may not be the same as being born small. However, particularly in developed countries, preterm births are responsible for a significant proportion of births less than 2.5kg making a major contribution to the overall birthweight distribution in these countries.[1] In this chapter, as in others in the book, a clear distinction will be made between evidence that relates to preterm births and that related directly to birthweight, and care will be taken to distinguish the effects of being born early from those of being born small.

Birthweight and mortality

Birthweight is the major determinant of neonatal and infant mortality.[1] Infant mortality by birthweight group for all infants born in England and Wales in 1999[2] shows that birthweight within the range 2.5 to 3.49kg is associated with an increased mortality risk although considerably less than for infants < 2.5kg. However, the population attributable risk is relatively high as this birthweight range (2.5–3.49) includes 53% of UK births compared with only 7.6% in the low birthweight range.[2] In the UK in 1999, 2212 infant deaths were recorded < 2.5kg and 918 in the range 2.5–3.49kg.

Early neonatal mortality (within the first week of life) shows a similar distribution by birthweight group. Table 1.1 is based on data from Sweden, Norway and Denmark in the 1970s.[3] Although mortality is likely to be lower in all groups as a consequence of advances in neonatal care, the data demonstrate the same pattern as that shown in Table 1.1 with a falling risk through the birthweight groups with the lowest risk in infants born between 3501–5000g. There is a slight upturn in risk in the very small group of infants born over 5000g. The paper reports a similar pattern of risk by birthweight group for Danish neonatal deaths (within the first month of life) in 1977.[3]

Table 1.1: Early neonatal mortality by birthweight group (%) in Norway (1975–76), Sweden (1973) and Denmark (1974)

Birthweight group (g)	Sweden 1973	Denmark 1974	Norway 1975–76
Under 1500	45.80	46.40	55.00
1501–2500	4.60	3.30	3.50
2501–3000	0.47	0.43	0.43
3001–3500	0.18	0.14	0.15
3501–5000	0.11	0.10	0.09*
> 5000	0.20	–	0.18

Source: Suagstad, p. 185.[3]
*Birthweight interval 3501–4500g.

Stillbirths show a strong relationship with birthweight. In a major Finnish cohort study of infants born in 1966, the rate of stillbirths was 377.1/1000 for infants < 1500g, 240.0/1000 for those 1500–1999g, 66.1/1000 for those 2000–2499g falling to 6.2/1000 for infants ⩾ 2500g.[4] More recent studies support the association of stillbirth with low birthweight[5] and small for gestational age (SGA) infants.[6] Late fetal deaths were greatly increased in extremely SGA fetuses (range 16 to 45 per 1000) compared with non-SGA fetuses (range 1.4 to 4.6 per 1000) in a study from Sweden.[7]

Draper *et al.*[8] report the survival to discharge from the neonatal unit by gestational age and birthweight of infants born between 22 to 32 weeks' gestation in the Trent Region of the UK. The delicate relationship between survival, birthweight and gestational age is demonstrated by the following survival patterns: at 24 weeks' gestation, survival ranged from 9% for infants of birthweight 250–499g to 21% for those of 1000–1249g; at 27 weeks' gestation, survival ranged from 55% for infants weighing 500–749g to 80% for those of 1250–1499g. For infants born at term, the relationship between survival and birthweight is also evident. Compared with infants born with weights over the 10th percentile, SGA infants (weights < 10th percentile) had a six times higher risk of perinatal death although the difference disappeared once infants who died with congenital malformations were excluded.[9] Among infants with major congenital malformations, birthweight and the number of malformations were the strongest risk factors for mortality within the first year of life.[10]

Advances in neonatal care have been associated with improvements in survival of low birthweight and preterm infants. Survival to one year of age of infants born less than 1000g in Sweden improved from less than 20% in 1973–75 to 50% in 1986–88.[11] For infants born between 1000 and 1499g, 90% survived in the 1986–88 cohort compared with 60% in the earlier cohort. A study from the UK Northern Region[12] reports improved survival between 1983 and 1994 for infants born less than 28 weeks' gestation.

Birthweight continues to exert an effect on mortality beyond the neonatal period and the first year of life. Sudden unexpected death in infancy is negatively associated with birthweight independent of gestational age.[13] In a population-based cohort study of 5914 Brazilian liveborn infants, the cumulative risk of death between one and four years of age was 21/1000 for infants weighing < 2000g at birth compared with 4/1000 for those weighing 3500g or more.[14] Survival to five years of age in an Indian cohort was better for normal birth-weight compared with low birthweight infants.[15] Finnish children born in 1966 had a cumulative risk of death between 28 days and 14 years that increased from 10.1/1000 for those with birthweight $\geqslant$ 2500g to 39.5/1000 for those < 1500g at birth.[4] The intermediate weight groups (1500–1999g and 2000–2499g) had rates of 21.1/1000 and 28.3/1000 respectively. Based on the Norwegian Birth Registry, Samuelsen *et al.* report relative risks, adjusted for gestational age, of 2.18 (95% confidence interval (CI) 1.85,2.56) of death from all causes at one to five years of age, 1.83 (95% CI 1.35,2.48) at 6–10 years and 1.35 (95% CI 0.91,1.99) at 11–15 years for children with birthweight < 2500g compared to those weighing 2500g or more.[16] However, analysis of the 1958 UK National Childhood Development Study cohort failed to show any significant increase in risk of death between 1–15 years for any birthweight groups less than those weighing 4250g or more despite showing a charac-teristic pattern of decreasing infant mortality with increasing birthweight.[17]

The relationship of birthweight with mortality beyond one year of age varies with cause of death. Among Norwegian children surviving the first year of life,[16] death from malformations showed a log-linear decrease in mortality with increasing birthweight while infection, accidents and other causes showed a J-shaped association with birthweight with a slight upturn in mortality in children who were very heavy at birth. Infectious disease mortality (one month to seven years) was increased in moderately low birthweight children from a hospital-based study in the USA but these authors report that the increased vulnerability is primarily attributable to preterm birth rather than intrauterine growth retardation.[18] Cancer deaths have been reported to show a positive relationship with birthweight (the opposite of its association with other causes of death) in the Norwegian study based on a whole country birth population between 1968–1991.[16] A case-control study from the USA reports a different pattern: girls aged one to ten years dying of solid tumours had a significantly higher mean birthweight independent of potential confounding factors but boys who died of solid tumours between birth and two years of age had a significantly lower mean birthweight.[19]

Birthweight and mortality

- Risk of stillbirth, neonatal death and infant death is inversely related to birthweight apart from a slight upturn in the risk in the small number of babies born $\geqslant 4500$g.
- Birthweight between 3500–4500g seems to be the optimal range for survival in the first year of life.
- Although gestational age is the more powerful determinant of mortality among infants < 2500g, birthweight, even below 2500g, has an effect on mortality independent of gestational age.
- A number of studies report an inverse relationship of birthweight to mortality in childhood beyond the age of 1 year independent of gestational age.
- Risk of death from cancer in childhood may be associated with higher birthweight.

Birthweight and neurodevelopmental, sensory and other disorders in childhood

Birthweight, mainly through its links with preterm birth, is strongly associated with risk of health problems in early infancy. The lower the infant's birthweight, the greater the likelihood of a prolonged stay in a neonatal unit after birth and of a range of problems, respiratory, vascular and neurological amongst others, related to being born too early or too small. These problems are not considered in detail here – those interested are referred to the extensive neonatology literature. Here the focus is on the longer term influences of birthweight in childhood some of which are linked to the infant's neonatal history. Among these influences, the most pervasive and significant are the effects on neurodevelopment and sensory functioning.

Disability (not defined by the authors) at ages 7 and 16 in males, and ages 7 and 23 in females, was reported to show a significant negative linear trend across birthweight groups in the National Child Development Study cohort.[17]

These trends remained following adjustment for gestational age. Using a broader definition of 'handicap including educational subnormality', Rantakallio and von Wendt[4] report a similar relationship with birthweight in 14-year-old Finnish children born in 1966.

Many studies chart the higher rates of disability in low birthweight and preterm infants.[20,21] Of the 64% of New Zealand children born less than 28 weeks' gestation and < 1500g who survived to age seven to eight years, 28% had some disability.[22] Ten per cent of Dutch children born at less than 32 weeks' gestation and/or birthweight < 1500g in 1983 were reported to have severe disability or handicap at 9–14 years.[23] Severe delayed development at 30 months (scores on the Bayley Mental and Psychomotor Developmental Indexes more than 3 standard deviations (SD) below the mean) was reported in 19% of UK and Ireland children born at or before 25 weeks completed gestation in 1995 and a further 11% had scores between 2 and 3 SDs below the mean.[24] Many of the children upon whom these studies were based were born in the early 1980s and their outcomes may not reflect improvements associated with more recent advances in neonatal intensive care. However, Tin *et al.* report that, for infants born less than 28 weeks' gestation in the north of England, rates of severe disability did not improve in the 12 years between 1983 and 1994 despite important advances in neonatal care.[12] A population-based study from New South Wales, Australia[25] reaches a similar conclusion.

Table 1.2 shows the relationship of birthweight to cerebral palsy in a cohort of 105 702 children born in the West Sussex Health Region of the UK between 1982 and 1996 (unpublished data). The pattern of very high rates below 1500g decreasing to a plateau between 3500–4500g is remarkably similar to the relationship of birthweight with infant mortality and early neonatal mortality shown in Table 1.1.

Table 1.2: Cerebral palsy prevalence by birthweight group in West Sussex, 1982–96

Birthweight group	Cerebral palsy	Without cerebral palsy	Rate/1000
< 1500g (n = 849)	55	794	64.7/1000
1500–1999g (n = 1386)	37	1349	26.6/1000
2000–2499g (n = 4192)	34	4158	8.1/1000
2500–2999g (n = 16942)	49	16893	2.9/1000
3000–3499g (n = 39143)	60	39083	1.5/1000
3500–3999g (n = 31692)	43	31649	1.3/1000
4000–4499g (n = 9939)	10	9929	1.0/1000
⩾ 4500g (n = 1559)	4	1555	2.6/1000

It should also be noted that, despite the greatly increased risk among infants < 2500g, low birthweight infants make up only 43% of all children with cerebral palsy compared with 37% among those with birthweights from 2500 to

3500g. As with mortality, the risk increases slightly for infants $\geqslant$ 4500g. This association of cerebral palsy with birthweight has been widely reported.[26,27,28] Norwegian cerebral palsy rates declined from 2.8/1000 in the five-year birth cohort born 1970–74 to 2.0/1000 in children born 1985–89 and birthweight specific cerebral palsy rates showed a declining trend in infants 500–1499g and infants weighing $\geqslant$ 2500g.[26] The authors suggest that this decline may be partly explained by a lower low birthweight rate (500–2499g) in the population in 1980–89 (3.8%) compared with 4.2% in 1970–79.

High rates of blindness and severe visual impairment, deafness and speech impairment have been described among low birthweight infants particularly those weighing 500–999g[29] and < 1250g.[30] Infants weighing less than 1250g at birth were more likely than those weighing between 1250–1999g to suffer major sensory impairments.[30] More subtle developmental and sensory impairments have been identified in more recent follow-up into adolescence among infants born < 1500g and/or before 28 weeks' gestation: impaired motor skills on the Motor Assessment Battery for Children;[31] increased tendency to left- or mixed-handedness;[32] reduced visual function with poor contrast sensitivity and strabismus.[33]

A range of other adverse health outcomes in childhood are associated with birthweight. Birthweight less than 1500g and preterm birth were associated with preschool asthma in a provincial health organisation in Canada.[34] Low birthweight was independently associated with episodes of wheezing by the age of five years but not at aged 16 years in the 1970 UK cohort study (Child Health and Education Study).[35] A more recent UK cohort (the Avon Longitudinal Study of Parents and Children) reports an association of concentrations of ferritin at 12 and 18 months of age with birthweight.[36] Lower birthweight appears to be associated with child abuse and neglect.[37] Rates of child abuse have been reported to increase with decreasing birthweight: in a study reported from Cardiff, rates increased from 2.1/1000 live births among infants weighing $\geqslant$ 3001g through 3.8/1000 among those weighing 2001–3000g to 13.0/1000 among those weighing 2000g or less.[38]

The association of birthweight with adverse health outcomes in childhood is reflected in an increased risk of hospital admission. Table 1.3 shows the proportion of infants in different birthweight groups admitted to hospital (including an overnight stay) for any cause by 8 weeks, 8 months, 18 months and 3 years in the Coventry Cohort Study (Spencer and Coe: unpublished data).

Looking down the columns, the familiar pattern of increasing risk of admission associated with decreasing birthweight group is evident up to 18 months but the association with decreasing birthweight group appears to be lost between 18 months and 3 years. Admissions for viral gastroenteritis between one month and one year of age in Washington State from 1987 to 1995 showed a similar pattern: with birthweight group 2500–4000g as reference, infants < 1500g

Table 1.3: Hospital admission at different ages in early childhood by birthweight group

Birthweight group	Hospital admission by 8 weeks (excluding neonatal admission) (%)	Hospital admission 8 weeks–8 months (%)	Hospital admission 8–18 months (%)	Hospital admission 18 months–3 years (%)
< 1500g	17.0	41.7	44.4	0
1500–1999g	15.4	23.3	13.8	5.0
2000–2499g	5.3	11.8	10.5	7.2
2500–2999g	4.8	11.9	11.6	11.5
3000–3499g	4.2	8.7	9.1	6.8
3500–3999g	2.4	8.0	8.5	6.9
4000–4499g	6.5	8.8	10.0	7.3
≥ 4500g	2.9	6.7	10.5	6.3

had a risk of admission of 2.6 (95% CI 1.6,4.1), those 1500–2499g a risk of 1.6 (95% CI 1.3,2.1) and those > 4000g were at reduced risk of 0.8 (95% CI 0.6,0.9).[39] Among a cohort of infants discharged from a New York Neonatal Intensive Care Unit, 6.4% of infants < 1500g at birth, 2.8% of those weighing 1500–2499g and 1.7% weighing > 2500g were readmitted with respiratory syncytial virus infection before three years of age.[40] Infants who were intrauterine growth retarded at birth had a two-fold increased risk of admission with diarrhoea before their second birthday compared with appropriate birthweight infants in a Brazilian birth cohort.[41] Preterm infants had only a slightly increased risk. Admission for pneumonia, however, was more likely in both intrauterine growth retarded and preterm infants. Based on the same cohort, the authors report an association between short, thin (low ponderal index) infants at birth and hospital admission from any cause in the first year of life.[42]

Birthweight and neurodevelopmental, sensory and other disorders

- Birthweight is strongly correlated with risk of disability in childhood.
- Risk of cerebral palsy shows a J-shaped relationship with birthweight: very low birthweight infants have a particularly high risk falling to a plateau between 4000–4500g with a slight rise in very heavy infants.
- Very low birthweight infants and those born less than 28 weeks' gestation are at high risk of major sensory impairments.
- More subtle motor and sensory impairments are also more common in very low birthweight and very preterm infants.
- Risk of hospital admission in early childhood shows a negative linear relationship with birthweight.

The influence of birthweight on cognitive function and educational attainment in childhood

Richards *et al.*[43] examined the effect of birthweight on cognitive function in the 1946 British birth cohort. The relationship of birthweight with cognitive function was examined at 8, 11, 15, 26 and 43 years in 3900 cohort members. After adjustment for gender, father's social class, mother's education and birth order, birthweight was significantly and positively associated with cognitive ability at ages 8, 11, 15 and 26 (*see* Table 1.4). Associations at 11, 15 and 23 were dependent on the association at eight.

Table 1.4: Cognitive function at 8, 11 and 23 years by birthweight group

Birthweight groups (kg)	Number of participants (%)	Adjusted mean differences (95% CI) in standardised cognitive score (3.01–3.50 as reference)
Age 8 years (n = 3773)		
0–2.50	174 (4.6)	−0.25 (−0.40,−0.12)
2.51–3.00	618 (16.4)	−0.06 (−0.15,0.02)
3.01–3.50	1319 (35.0)	Reference
3.51–4.00	1242 (32.9)	0.16 (0.09,0.23)
4.01–5.00	420 (11.1)	0.18 (0.08,0.28)
Age 11 years (n = 3527)		
0–2.50	155 (4.4)	−0.21 (−0.12,0.07)
2.51–3.00	586 (16.6)	−0.09 (−0.17,0.00)
3.01–3.50	1233 (35.0)	Reference
3.51–4.00	1159 (32.9)	0.11 (0.04,0.18)
4.01–5.00	394 (11.2)	0.08 (−0.02,0.18)
Age 15 years (n = 3383)		
0–2.50	151 (4.5)	−0.24 (−0.39,−0.10)
2.51– 3.00	564 (16.7)	−0.12(−0.20,−0.03)
3.01–3.50	1174 (34.7)	Reference
3.51–4.00	1117 (33.0)	0.06 (−0.01,0.13)
4.01–5.00	337 (11.1)	0.08 (−0.02,0.18)
Age 23 years (n = 2888)		
0–2.50	135 (4.7)	−0.24 (−0.40,−0.08)
2.51–3.00	471 (16.3)	−0.09 (−0.18,0.01)
3.01–3.50	1006 (34.8)	Reference
3.51–4.00	966 (33.5)	0.06 (−0.02,0.14)
4.01–5.00	310 (10.7)	0.09 (−0.03,0.20)

Source: Richards *et al.*, p. 201.[43]

The authors also report a significant effect of birthweight on education with increasing birthweight being associated with higher educational attainment.

Similar results were reported from a study in 12 US cities.[44] The study sample was limited to children born at $\geq$ 37 weeks' gestation with birthweights 1500–3999g. Mean IQ at seven years of age increased monotonically with birthweight in both sexes across the range of birthweight following adjustment for maternal age, 'race', education, socio-economic status, and birth order. An historic Scottish cohort born in 1921 and studied at the age of 11 years[45] showed the same relationship of birthweight with cognitive function as did Danish conscripts aged 18 studied between 1973 and 1975.[46] In the Danish study, cognitive function decreased slightly above 4200g birthweight suggesting a J-shaped relationship with birthweight. Children born < 2500g had a higher risk of mild mental retardation odds ratio (OR) 2.4 (95% CI 1.6,3.8)) and severe mental retardation (OR 4.4 (95% CI 2.6,7.5)) in a case-control study of 10-year-olds in Atlanta, USA.[47] Very low birthweight infants had much higher risks of mild and severe mental retardation. In a survey of 9996 US children aged 7–17 years in 1988, low birthweight was associated with repeating kindergarten or first grade at school independent of confounding variables.[48] A range of studies have documented impairments of cognitive functioning and educational difficulties among very low birthweight and very preterm infants.[22,24,25,29,30,49–51] These infants have lower mean IQ scores and are more likely to require special education. Subtle educational difficulties such as reductions in reading performance[49] and cognitive problems such as everyday memory difficulties[52] are more common in these infants.

The impact of birthweight on cognitive functioning and educational attainment

- Cognitive functioning measured at various times in childhood shows a positive linear relationship with birthweight.
- One study suggests that this relationship may be J-shaped with a slight upturn in cognitive impairment above 4200g.
- Cognitive functioning and educational attainment are particularly impaired among infants born very low birthweight and/or very early – these infants frequently suffer subtle impairments that may not be readily detectable.

Factors that modify the effects of birthweight on childhood health outcomes

Although low birthweight infants are more likely to be born into households with adverse social conditions (*see* Chapter 5),[53,54] the social environment in which they live can modify the negative effects associated with being born small and/or early. Longitudinal data based on a cohort of Hawaiian children indicate that social environment is more predictive of poor child health outcome than low birthweight itself.[55] In a sample of 8661 US children aged 2 to 11 included in the 1981 Child Health Supplement of the National Health Interview Survey low birthweight (< 2500g) children were more likely to have worse outcomes when exposed to a high-risk social environment than similar 'normal' birthweight (≥ 2500g) children.[54] However, low birthweight children were no more likely than those of 'normal' birthweight to have poor health outcomes in either a low- or moderate-risk social environment (*see* Table 1.5).

Table 1.5: Influence of social environment on adverse outcomes associated with low birthweight

Outcome	Low-risk social environment		Moderate-risk social environment		High-risk social environment	
	NBW* (2156)	LBW** (142)	NBW (3753)	LBW (291)	NBW (2076)	LBW (243)
Bed days	24%	15%	48%	35%	28%	50%
School-loss days	22%	18%	45%	43%	33%	39%
Restricted activity days	27%	18%	48%	48%	25%	34%
School failure	26%	22%	49%	44%	25%	34%
Low school ranking	8%	15%	47%	36%	45%	49%
Behaviour problems	16%	10%	48%	33%	36%	56%
Maternal perception of child health as fair/poor	13%	12%	38%	32%	48%	56%

*'Normal' birthweight (NBW).
**Low birthweight (LBW).
Source: McGauhey *et al*.[54]

A study of very low birthweight infants from The Netherlands followed to the age of 3.6 years reports similar findings.[56] The authors conclude that children at high biological risk were able to catch up on their cognitive delay in a highly stimulating home environment and that children at low as well as high biological risk in a less stimulating home environment showed a decline in cognitive development. A study from Israel reports a significant protective effect of high socio-economic status on growth independent of birthweight.[57]

Definitions of ethnicity and 'race' are problematic and their effects on child health outcomes are difficult to disentangle from those of socio-economic factors.[58] However, various studies suggest that mortality rates in similar birthweight groups may be lower in some ethnic groups compared with others.[1,59–61] Infants born to mothers of Indian sub-continental origin in Blackburn in northern England had lower birthweight specific neonatal mortality for causes other than congenital malformations than infants born to mothers from elsewhere: in the birthweight group < 1000g they had a neonatal mortality rate (NMR) of 250/1000 compared with 516.1/1000 for other ethnic groups.[61] Infants of Indian sub-continental origin also had lower rates of assisted ventilation within each birthweight group. In a study based on births in a London borough, among those infants born alive from 28–36 weeks' gestation, black infants had lower neonatal death rates (7.7/1000) than white infants (19/1000).[62] Ethnicity has also been reported to have an effect independent of other factors on hospital admission in the first year of life in very preterm infants,[63] and growth of low birthweight infants up to two to three years of age.[64]

The above studies indicate that the impact of birthweight on some child health outcomes is likely to be modified or attentuated by the social environment in which the child is reared and some unknown aspect of ethnicity may protect against mortality at lower birthweights and gestational ages as well as some later adverse childhood outcomes associated with birthweight.

Chapter summary

- Birthweight is a major determinant of mortality in infancy and child-hood and of disability, cognitive functioning and other childhood health outcomes.

- The increased risk of death, disability, cognitive impairment and hospital admission associated with birthweight is not confined to low birth-weight infants but continues into the 'normal' birthweight range.

- There is evidence of a J-shaped relationship of birthweight with some childhood outcomes – infants born in the highest birthweight group are at slightly increased risk of death, disability and possibly cognitive impairment.

- Aspects of the social environment and possibly genetic and/or cultural factors seem to provide some protection for children against some of the adverse consequences of low birthweight.

References

1 Paneth N (1995) The problem of low birth weight. *The Future of Children.* **5**: 20–32.

2 Department of Health (2000) Perinatal and infant mortality statistics 1999. DH3, No. 32. Accessed at: www.statistics.gov.uk/downloads/theme_health/DH3No32book/Table14 on 29.7.02.

3 Suagstad LF (1981) Weight of all births and infant mortality. *J Epidemiol and Community Health.* **35**: 185–91.

4 Rantakallio P and von Wendt L (1985) Prognosis for low birthweight infants up to the age of 14: a population study. *Dev Med and Child Neurol.* **27**: 655–63.

5 Sheiner E, Hallak M, Shoham-Vardi I, Goldstein D, Mazor M and Katz M (2000) Determining risk factors for intrapartum fetal death. *J Repro Med.* **45**: 419–24.

6 Gardosi J, Mul T, Mongelli M and Fagan D (1998) Analysis of birthweight and gestational age in antepartum stillbirths. *Br J Obstetr and Gynaecol.* **105**: 524–30.

7 Cnattingius S, Haglund B and Kramer MS (1998) Differences in late fetal death rates in association with determinants of small for gestational age fetuses: population based cohort study. *BMJ.* **316**: 1483–7.

8 Draper ES, Manktelow B, Field DJ and James D (1999) Prediction of survival for preterm births by weight and gestational age: retrospective population based study. *BMJ.* **319**: 1093–7.

9 Vik T, Markestad T, Ahlsten G, GebreMedhin M, Jacobsen G, Hoffman HJ and Bakketeig LS (1997) Body proportions and early neonatal death in small-for-gestational age infants of successive births. *Acta Obstetr et Gynecol Scand.* **76**: 76–81.

10 Druschel C, Hughes JP and Olsen C (1996) Mortality among infants with congenital malformations, New York State, 1983 to 1988. *Public Health Reports.* **111**: 359–65.

11 Ericson A, Gunnarskog J, Kallen B and Olausson PO (1992) A registry study of very low birth weight liveborn infants in Sweden, 1973–1988. *Acta Obstetr et Gynecol Scand.* **71**: 104–11.

12 Tin W, Wariyar U and Hey E (1997) Changing prognosis for babies of less than 28 weeks' gestation in the north of England between 1983 and 1994. *BMJ.* **314**: 107–11.

13 Fleming P, Blair P, Bacon C and Berry J (eds) (2000) *Sudden Unexpected Death in Infancy: The CESDI SUDI Studies.* The Stationery Office, London: p. 25.

14 Victora CG, Barros FC, Huttly SR, Teixeira AM and Vaughan JP (1992) Early childhood mortality in a Brazilian cohort: the roles of birthweight and socioeconomic status. *Int J Epidemiol.* **21**: 911–5.

15 Hirve S and Ganatra B (1997) A prospective cohort study on the survival experience of under five children in rural western India. *Indian Pediatrics.* **34**: 995–1001.

16 Samuelsen SO, Magnus P and Bakketeig LS (1998) Birthweight and mortality in childhood in Norway. *Am J Epidemiol.* **148**: 983–91.

17 Power C and Li L (2000) Cohort study of birthweight, mortality and disability. *BMJ.* **320**: 840–1.

18 Read JS, Clemens JD and Klebanoff MA (1994) Moderate low birth weight and infectious disease mortality during infancy and childhood. *Am J Epidemiol.* **140**: 721–33.

19 Eisenberg DE and Sorahan T (1987) Birth weight and childhood cancer deaths. *J Nat Cancer Inst.* **78**: 1095–100.

20 Stewart AL, Reynolds EOR and Lipscomb AP (1981) Outcome for infants of very low birthweight: survey of world literature. *Lancet.* **i**: 1038–40.

21 Pharoah POD, Stevenson CJ, Cooke RWI and Stevenson RC (1994) Clinical and subclinical deficits at 8 years in a geographically defined cohort of low birthweight infants. *Arch Disease in Childhood.* **70**: 264–70.

22 Darlow BA, Horwood LJ, Mogridge N and Clemett RS (1998) Survival and disability at 7–8 years in New Zealand infants less than 28 weeks gestation. *NZ Med J.* **111**: 264–7.

23 Walther FJ, den Ouden AL and Verloove-Vanhorick SP (2000) Looking back in time: outcome of a national cohort of very preterm infants born in The Netherlands in 1983. *Early Human Development.* **59**: 175–91.

24 Wood NS, Marlow N, Costeloe K, Gibson AT and Wilkinson AR (2000) Neurologic and developmental disability after extremely preterm birth. EPICure Study Group. *NEJM.* **343**: 378–84.

25 Sutton L, Bajuk B and the New South Wales Neonatal Intensive Care Unit Study Group (1999) Population-based study of infants born at less than 28 weeks' gestation in New South Wales, Australia, in 1992–3. *Paed and Perinatal Epidemiol.* **13**: 288–301.

26 Meberg A and Broch H (1995) A changing pattern of cerebral palsy – declining trend for incidence of cerebral palsy in the 20 year period 1970–89. *J Perinatal Med.* **23**: 395–402.

27 Pharoah POD, Cooke T, Johnson MA, King R and Mutch L (1998) Epidemiology of cerebral palsy in England and Scotland, 1984–9. *Arch Disease in Childhood.* **79**: Fetal and Neonatal Edition F21–5.

28 Petridou E, Koussouri M, Toupadaki N, Papavassiliou A, Youroukos S, Katsarou E and Trichopoulos D (1996) Risk factors for cerebral palsy: a case-control study in Greece. *Scand J Soc Med.* **24**: 14–26.

29 Doyle LW, Casalaz D for the Victorian Infant Collaborative Study Group (2001) Outcome at 14 years of extremely low birthweight infants: a regional study. *Arch Disease in Childhood.* **85**: Fetal and Neonatal Edition F159–64.

30 Marlow N, D'Souza SW and Chiswick ML (1987) Neurodevelopmental outcome in babies weighing less than 2001g at birth. *BMJ.* **294**: Clinical Research Edition 1582–6.

31 Powls A, Botting N, Cooke RW and Marlow N (1995) Motor impairment in children 12–13 years old with a birthweight of less than 1250g. *Arch Disease in Childhood.* **73**: Fetal and Neonatal Edition F62–6.

32 Powls A, Botting N, Cooke RW and Marlow N (1996) Handedness in very low birthweight (VLBW) children at 12 years of age: relation to perinatal and outcome variables. *Dev Med and Child Neurol.* **38**: 594–602.

33 Powls A, Botting N, Cooke RW, Stephenson G and Marlow N (1997) Visual impairment in very low birthweight children. *Arch Disease in Childhood.* **76**: Fetal and Neonatal Edition F82–7.

34 Schaubel D, Johansen H, Dutta M, Desmeules M and Becker AM (1996) Neonatal characteristics as risk factors for preschool asthma. *J Asthma.* **33**: 255–64.

35 Lewis S, Richards D, Bynner J, Butler N and Britton J (1995) Prospective study of risk factors for early and persistent wheezing in childhood. *Eur Resp J.* **8**: 349–56.

36 Sherriff A, Emond A, Hawkins N and Golding J (1999) Haemoglobin and ferritin concentrations in children aged 12 and 18 months. ALSPAC Children in Focus Study Team. *Arch Disease in Childhood.* **80**: 153–7.

37 Schloesser P, Pierpont J and Poertner J (1992) Active surveillance of child abuse fatalities. *Child Abuse and Neglect.* **16**: 3–10.

38 Murphy JF, Jenkins J, Newcombe RG and Sibert JR (1981) Objective birth data and the prediction of child abuse. *Arch Disease in Childhood.* **56**: 295–7.

39 Newman RD, Grupp-Phelan J, Shay DK and Davis RL (1999) Perinatal risk factors for infant hospitalization with viral gastroenteritis. *Pediatrics.* **103**: E3.

40 Nachman SA, Navaie-Waliser M and Qureshi MZ (1997) Rehospitalization with respiratory syncytial virus after neonatal intensive care unit discharge: a 3-year follow up. *Pediatrics.* **100**: E8.

41 Barros FC, Huttly SR, Victora CG, Kirkwood BR and Vaughan JP (1992) Comparison of the causes and consequences of prematurity and intrauterine growth retardation: a longitudinal study in southern Brazil. *Pediatrics.* **90**: 238–44.

42 Morris SS, Victora CG, Barros FC, Halpern R, Menezes AM, Cesar JA, Horta BL and Tomasi E (1998) Length and ponderal index at birth: associations with mortality, hospitalizations, development and post-natal growth in Brazilian infants. *Int J Epidemiol.* **27**: 242–7.

43 Richards M, Hardy R, Kuh D and Wadsworth MEJ (2001) Birth weight and cognitive function in the British 1946 birth cohort: longitudinal population based study. *BMJ.* **322**: 199–203.

44 Matte TD, Bresnahan M, Begg MD and Susser E (2001) Influence of variation in birth weight within normal range and within sibships on IQ at age 7 years: cohort study. *BMJ.* **323**: 310–4.

45 Shenkin SD, Starr JM, Pattie A, Rush MA, Whalley LJ and Deary IJ (2001) Birth weight and cognitive function at age 11 years: the Scottish Mental Survey 1932. *Arch Disease in Childhood.* **85**: 189–97.

46 Sørensen HT, Sabroe S, Olson J, Rothman KJ, Gillman MW and Fischer P (1997) Birth weight and cognitive function in young adult life: historical cohort study. *BMJ.* **315**: 401–3.

47 Mervis CA, Decouflé P, Murphy CC and Yeargin-Allsopp M (1995) Low birthweight and the risk for mental retardation later in childhood. *Paed and Perinatal Epidemiol.* **9**: 455–68.

48 Byrd RS and Weitzman ML (1994) Predictors of early grade retention among children in the United States. *Pediatrics.* **93**: 481–7.

49 Marlow N, Roberts L and Cooke R (1993) Outcome at 8 years for children with birth weights of 1250g or less. *Arch Disease in Childhood.* **68**: 286–90.

50 Botting N, Powls A, Cooke RW and Marlow N (1998) Cognitive and educational outcome of very low birthweight children in early adolescence. *Dev Med and Child Neurol.* **40**: 652–60.

51 Aylward GP, Pfeiffer SI, Wright A and Vershulst SJ (1989) Outcome of studies of low birth weight infants published in the last decade. *J Pediatrics.* **115**: 515–20.

52 Briscoe J, Gathercole Se and Marlow N (2001) Everyday memory and cognitive ability in children born very prematurely. *J Child Psychol and Psychiatry.* **42**: 749–54.

53 Kramer MS, Séguin L, Lydon J and Goulet L (2000) Socio-economic disparities in pregnancy outcome: why do the poor fare so poorly? *Paed and Perinatal Epidemiol.* **14**: 194–210.

54 McGauhey PJ, Starfield B, Alexander C and Ensmiger ME (1991) Social environment and vulnerability of low birth weight children: a social-epidemiological perspective. *Pediatrics.* **88**: 943–53.

55 Werner EE and Smith RS (1982) *Vulnerable But Invincible: a longitudinal study of resilient children and youth.* McGraw-Hill, New York.

56 Weisglas-Kuperus N, Baerts W, Smrkovsky M and Sauer PJJ (1993) Effects of biological and social factors on the cognitive development of very low birth weight children. *Pediatrics.* **92**: 658–65.

57 Diamond G, Zalzberg J, Inbar D, Cohen Z, Kaks Y, Geva D, Grossman T and Cohen HJ (2001) Birth order, birth weight and later patterns of growth. *Ambulatory Child Health.* **7**: 259–68.

58 Spencer NJ (1996) Race and ethnicity as determinants of child health: a personal view. *Child: Care, Health and Development.* **22**: 327–46.

59 Wilcox A and Russell IT (1990) Why small black infants have a lower mortality than small white infants: the case for population-specific standards for birth weight. *J Pediatrics.* **116**: 7–10.

60 Dawson I, Golder RY and Jonas EG (1982) Birthweight by gestational age and its effect on perinatal mortality in white and Punjabi births. *Br J Obstetr and Gynaecol.* **89**: 896–9.

61 Jivani SK (1986) Asian neonatal mortality in Blackburn. *Arch Disease in Childhood.* **61**: 510–2.

62 Lyon AJ, Clarkson P, Jeffrey I and West GA (1994) Effect of ethnic origin of mother on fetal outcome. *Archives of Disease in Childhood.* **70**: F40–3.

63 Elder DE, Hagan R, Evans SF, Benninger HR and French NP (1999) Hospital admission in the first year of life in very preterm infants. *J Paed and Child Health.* **35**: 145–50.

64 Seed PT, Ogundipe EM and Wolfe CDA (2000) Ethnic differences in the growth of low-birthweight infants. *Paed Perinatal Epidem.* **14**: 4–13.

CHAPTER 2

Birthweight and health in adulthood

The second chapter in Part 1 deals with the impact of birthweight on adult health. Interest in the antecedents of adult disease goes back as far as the beginning of the 20th century[1] but it was not until the 1970s that interest in the potential role of fetal growth and birthweight in adult disease developed as a result of the studies linking birthweight to cardiovascular mortality and morbidity in adulthood.[2] Based on these studies, Barker developed the fetal programming hypothesis otherwise known as the Barker hypothesis.[2,3] As the focus of this chapter is the evidence linking birthweight with a range of adult health outcomes, the competing explanations and hypotheses[4,5] for these associations will be discussed only in so far as they throw light on this relationship.

The impact of birthweight on death from cardiovascular disease (CVD) is considered first, followed by the evidence for links with cardiovascular morbidity and risk factors for heart disease including blood pressure and obesity. Impaired glucose tolerance (IGT) and non-insulin dependent diabetes mellitus (NIDDM) and their links with birthweight are discussed next. The evidence linking birthweight through childhood respiratory illness to adult respiratory disease is presented. Cancer in adulthood has also been linked to fetal and early childhood growth; the links are discussed in relation to different types of cancer. Height attained and cognitive functioning in adults have been associated with birthweight. The evidence for these associations is considered.

Finally, in view of the close association of birthweight with socio-economic status (SES) (*see* Chapter 5) and the possible role of social factors in mediating birthweight's impact on adult health, the links between childhood SES and adult health will be reviewed briefly.

Birthweight and cardiovascular mortality, morbidity and cardiac risk factors in adulthood

Based on a cohort of men and women born in Hertfordshire, England between 1911 and 1930, a decline in mortality risk from coronary heart disease with increasing birthweight in men and women with a slight increase in risk in the heaviest birthweight group was noted (*see* Table 2.1).[6]

Table 2.1: Coronary health disease mortality by birthweight group among men born 1911–30 and women born 1923–30

Birthweight (lb)	Rate ratios for coronary heart disease mortality: Men (born 1911–30)	Rate ratios for coronary heart disease mortality: Women (born 1923–30)
≤ 5.5	1.00	1.00
–6	0.81	0.87
–7	0.80	0.81
–8	0.74	0.71
–9	0.55	0.52
≥ 10	0.65	0.59
p-value for trend	p < 0.0005	not specified

Source: Osmond *et al*.[6]

The Hertfordshire findings, showing the same J-shaped relationship with birthweight seen in many childhood health outcomes (*see* Chapter 1), were initially replicated in a study of singleton men born in Sheffield between 1907 and 1924.[7] Subsequently there have been many studies confirming this relationship from a range of different countries.[8–10] Mortality from cerebrovascular disease has also been shown to have the same relationship with birthweight.[11,12]

Non-fatal CVD has been shown to have the same reverse J-shaped relationship with self-reported birthweight among women aged 46–71 in 1992 enrolled in the US Nurses' Health Study (*see* Figure 2.1).[13] Among middle-aged men from Caerphilly in south Wales, a reverse relationship was found with non-fatal myocardial infarction.[14]

Raised blood pressure and obesity are important markers of cardiovascular risk. However, their relationship with birthweight is not so clear. Among children aged 9–11 years an inverse relationship of both systolic and diastolic blood pressure with low birthweight was noted after adjustment for age, sex, height and body mass index (BMI) (*see* Figure 2.2).[15]

An inverse association of systolic blood pressure with birthweight was also noted in a study of Jamaican school children aged 6–16 years.[16] Interestingly, although studies have also shown the same relationship in adulthood[14,17–20] and a tracking effect of blood pressure has been noted from childhood through into adult life,[21] two studies in adolescence fail to show the expected inverse relationship with blood pressure.[22,23]

The relationship of birthweight with adult obesity is disputed. Birthweight was reported to be positively rather than negatively associated with BMI in Danish men aged 18–26 years[24] and in late adolescence in a US study.[25] Others

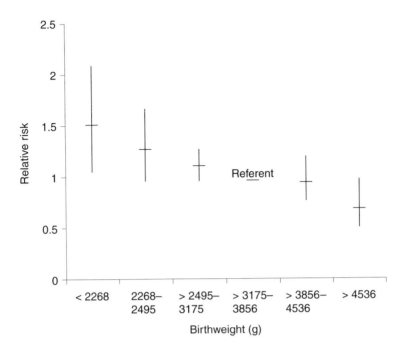

Figure 2.1: Relative risks with 95% CIs for non-fatal CVD by birthweight.

Source: Frankel *et al.*[14]

have shown a negative relationship[26] but there remains an apparent paradox – hypertension and obesity are well recognised and closely associated risk factors for CVD but their associations with birthweight are less clear and, in the case of obesity, they may be in the opposite direction from that expected. Various explanations have been advanced for this paradox: the risk factors for obesity and CVD may operate through different causal pathways;[24] impaired fetal growth, expressed as lower birthweight and thinness at birth, may be associated with a propensity to develop high blood pressure that is only fully expressed among those who become obese in later life.[20]

A further interesting possibility raised by a study based on the Avon Longitudinal Study of Parents and Children (ALSPAC)[27] is that infants with lower weight, length and ponderal index at birth who show catch-up growth in early childhood may constitute a high risk group for both adult obesity and CVD in adulthood. This would be consistent with the so-called 'thrifty phenotype' hypothesis advanced by Hales and Barker[28] to explain the relationship of poor fetal growth with non-insulin dependent diabetes (*see below*). In essence, this hypothesis suggests that fetal cells programmed by poor nutrition at critical

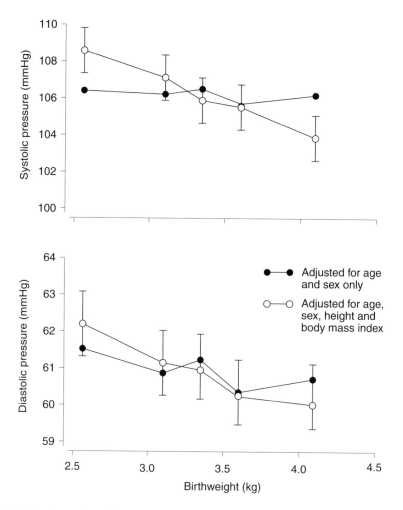

Figure 2.2: Birthweight and blood pressure at 9–11 years, showing effect of adjustment for current body size. Mean blood pressures and 95% CIs (bars) are shown for each fifth of birthweight.

periods of fetal life are unable to cope with abundant nutrition in childhood or adult life. Thus, infants with lower weights at birth subsequently exposed to abundant nutrition and becoming obese adults may constitute a particularly high risk group for high blood pressure and CVD. It is also consistent with the finding that abdominal fat storage, known to increase the risk of CVD independently of obesity, may be a persisting response to adverse conditions and growth failure in fetal life and infancy.[29]

Birthweight and cardiovascular mortality, morbidity and risk factors in adult life

- Mortality from coronary heart disease and cerebrovascular disease in adult life shows a J-shaped relationship with birthweight.
- A similar relationship has been reported with non-fatal coronary disease in men and women.
- There is strong evidence for an association of blood pressure in childhood and adulthood with birthweight despite two studies that failed to show an association in adolescence.
- Birthweight appears to be positively associated with adult obesity – however, this paradox may be partly explained by an association of low birthweight with increased abdominal fat storage which is known to increase cardiovascular risk independent of obesity.

Birthweight and non-insulin dependent diabetes mellitus and impaired glucose tolerance

In a sub-sample of the Hertfordshire cohort (*see above*) still resident in the county, a clear linear relationship was demonstrated between diabetes or impaired glucose tolerance and birthweight (Table 2.2).[30]

Table 2.2: Odds of high two hour glucose concentration adjusted for BMI by birthweight group

Birthweight group (lb)	(g)	Odds ratio for two hour glucose concentration of $\geqslant$ 7.8mmol/l adjusted for BMI (95% CI)
$\leqslant$ 5.5	$\leqslant$ 2495 (n = 20)	6.6 (1.5,28)
–6.5	–2948 (n = 47)	4.8 (1.3,17)
–7.5	–3402 (n = 104)	4.6 (1.4,16)
–8.5	–3856 (n = 117)	2.6 (0.8,8.9)
–9.5	–4309 (n = 54)	1.4 (0.3,5.6)
> 9.5	> 4309 (n = 28)	1.0 (reference)
χ^2 for linear trend		15.4 (p < 0.001)

Source: Hales *et al.*, p. 244.[30]

Subsequent reports confirm the relationship of birthweight with diabetes or impaired glucose tolerance although not all show the same linear relationship. Among 266 men and women born in a hospital in Preston and studied at a mean age of 50 years, a linear relationship of birthweight to new NIDDM or IGT was demonstrated.[31] Among US male health professionals studied at a mean age of 61 years, with the birthweight group 3.2–3.8kg as reference, the odds ratio for NIDDM was 1.9 in those in the lowest birthweight group (< 2.5kg) and 1.4 in the birthweight group 2.5–3.1kg.[32] No trend in NIDDM prevalence was found at the higher levels of birthweight. A stepwise increase in NIDDM prevalence among 60 year old men living in Uppsala was noted in those in the lowest birthweight category (< 3.25kg).[33] However, this association only reached statistical significance when adjustment was made for BMI. A study among Pima Native Americans, a population with a high incidence of diabetes, reported a U-shaped relationship between birthweight and prevalence of diabetes. Prevalence was raised only in those with birthweights < 2.5kg or > 4.5kg.[34] The authors suggest an alternative hypothesis to the thrifty phenotype (*see above*). They suggest that the increase in prevalence of diabetes among low birthweight subjects could reflect the selective survival of low birthweight infants genetically susceptible to developing diabetes.

Birthweight and non-insulin dependent diabetes mellitus and impaired glucose tolerance

- There is good evidence of an association of birthweight with NIDDM and impaired glucose tolerance in adult life although the exact relationship has been shown to be different in different populations.
- In northern European populations the relationship is either linear or showing a stepwise increase up to 3.25kg.

Birthweight and respiratory illness and cancer in adulthood

Results from the British 1948 national cohort study (the MRC National Survey of Health and Development)[35] show that low birthweight, along with living in crowded home circumstances at two years of age and a parental history of bronchitis, was independently associated with reduced peak expiratory flow rate at 36 years of age even after adjustment for smoking, education and adult socio-economic circumstances. Forced expiratory volume in one second (FEV 1) measured at 35 years of age in the British 1958 national cohort study was positively related to birthweight (after exclusion of those born preterm) after adjustment for adult height, smoking and SES in childhood and adult life.[36]

Based on the Hertfordshire cohort, Barker *et al.*[37] showed a weak trend of falling standardised mortality ratios (SMR) for chronic obstructive airways disease with increasing birthweight. The numbers of deaths were small making interpretation difficult but there was a striking difference between the SMR for men with birthweights $\leqslant$ 5.5lb (SMR 131) and those with birthweights $>$ 9.5lb

(SMR 28). This paper also reported a linear relationship between FEV 1 and birthweight (*see* Table 2.3). This relationship persisted after adjustment for current height, age, smoking and social class.

Table 2.3: Mean forced expiratory volume (FEV 1) in men by birthweight group

Birthweight (lb)	Number of men	Mean forced expiratory volume at one second adjusted for height and age
≤ 5.5	33	2.28
−6.5	103	2.41
−7.5	258	2.44
−8.5	242	2.52
−9.5	132	2.55
> 9.5	57	2.57

Source: Barker *et al.*, p. 154.[37]

The results of this study failed to show any trend in SMRs for lung cancer by birthweight. Other studies show an inconsistent relationship of birthweight with cancer in adult life. Stomach cancer is likely to be linked with birthweight through the association of both with lower SES.[38] A Swedish case-control study failed to show any gradient of breast cancer with birthweight[39] but another study suggests a positive relationship between birthweight and breast cancer.[40] An increased risk of testicular cancer with impaired fetal growth has been reported in two studies[41,42] but a more recent study reports a J-shaped relationship with those weighing < 2.5kg having an OR of 2.59 (95% CI 1.05,6.38) and those weighing > 3.99kg an OR of 1.58 (95% CI 1.10,2.29) compared with a reference group weighing 2.5–3.99kg.[43] Prostatic cancer has also been associated with birthweight but in this case the association is with high birthweight.[44]

Birthweight and respiratory illness and cancer in adulthood

- A weak linear relationship of birthweight with death from chronic obstructive lung disease has been reported.
- Lung function (peak expiratory flow and FEV 1) in adult life is associated with birthweight independent of confounding variables such as smoking.
- The relationship of birthweight with adult cancer is unclear – there is some evidence linking higher birthweight with breast cancer and cancer of the prostate.

Birthweight and attained height and cognitive function in adulthood

Attained height is associated with risk of subsequent adult health outcomes. Short stature increases the risk of adverse pregnancy outcome,[45] mortality from coronary heart disease[46] and obstructive lung disease.[47] Counties of England and Wales with taller populations have been shown to have lower mortality from chronic bronchitis, rheumatic heart disease, ischaemic heart disease and stroke, and higher mortality from breast, prostate and ovarian cancer.[48]

In a large study from Israel (30 083 subjects born in Jerusalem between 1964 and 1971), a significant increase in standing height at age 17 by birthweight of 3.33cm/1000g was reported for males and 2.85cm/1000g for females.[49] This relationship persisted after adjustment for social class and ethnic origin. Birthweight was associated with adult height in the British 1948 cohort independent of other confounding variables such as social class, sex and parental height.[35] A similar association was noted in the British 1958 national cohort.[50] A cohort study from France demonstrated a reduction in height at 20 years of age of 4.5cm in men and 3.94cm in women born small for gestational age (SGA) compared with normal for gestational age subjects.[51] Another study reported a seven-fold higher risk of short stature among young adults who were small for gestational age compared with normal for gestational age subjects.[52]

Another factor that has been shown to have an impact on adult health outcomes is education which in turn is affected by cognitive function. The association of birthweight with cognitive function and educational achievement in childhood was discussed in Chapter 1. Here, the evidence for an effect of birthweight extending into adulthood is considered. Although there is reasonable evidence for a link between cognitive function and birthweight in childhood, results of studies extending in adulthood are conflicting. The study of Danish conscripts,[53] already discussed in Chapter 1, reports a J-shaped relationship with birthweight. Members of the British 1946 cohort studied at aged 43 (*see also* Chapter 1) continued to demonstrate a weak association of birthweight with cognitive function after adjustment for sex, father's social class, mother's education and birth order.[54] These findings suggest that the association with birthweight may dissipate with increasing age. This would be consistent with the findings among older men and women[55] who had been born in Hertfordshire, Preston and Sheffield between 1920 and 1943 that failed to show any consistent association between impaired fetal growth and cognitive function. SGA subjects who were part of the British 1970 national cohort showed significant differences in academic achievement and professional attainment at 26 years of age compared with normal birthweight subjects.[56] However, the author reports no long-term social or emotional consequences of being SGA.

Birthweight and attained height and cognitive function in adulthood

- There is strong evidence of a positive linear relationship of height attained with birthweight.
- The relationship of birthweight with cognitive function in adult life is less clear – the evidence suggests that the linear relationship noted in childhood and early adulthood may weaken and possibly disappear in later life.

Childhood socio-economic status and adult health

The social patterning of birthweight is well recognised (*see* Chapter 5) and birthweight has been shown to be associated with later socio-economic disadvantage.[57] Data from the British 1958 national cohort demonstrate a linear trend in financial difficulties experienced at least once by the age of 23 years with decreasing birthweight such that 39.2% of the lowest birthweight quintile experienced difficulties compared with 31.6% of the highest quintile.[57] These data suggest that socio-economic circumstances throughout the life course and especially in childhood may be important in understanding the impact of birthweight on adult health. For this reason, this section briefly reviews the evidence for the impact of childhood SES on adult health and the potential pathways by which birthweight and early SES might combine to influence adult health outcomes.

Forsdahl[58] was among the first to suggest a link between poor living conditions in childhood and adolescence and mortality from coronary heart disease. Subsequently, links have been reported between poor social circumstances in childhood and a range of adult health outcomes: all cause mortality among males;[59] mortality among men and women with chronic illnesses by 36 years of age;[60] physiological risk factors for CVD (serum cholesterol, blood pressure, body mass index and FEV 1);[61] chronic obstructive airways disease and reduced peak expiratory flow rate at 36 years of age;[35] short stature;[50,62] obesity;[63] limiting longstanding illness;[64,65] self-reported poor health.[50,65] Lundberg,[66] whilst confirming an association of childhood economic conditions with self-reported ill health, suggests that family conflicts may be more important than economic conditions in determining adult mortality and physical and mental health.

It is interesting to note that the adult health conditions linked to poor socio-economic circumstances are similar to those linked to birthweight (*see above*). Lamont *et al.*,[67] in discussing the methodology for their planned examination of adult health outcomes among members of the Newcastle Thousand Families study,[68] propose a model of the relationships between early life and later experience and adult disease risk (*see* Figure 2.3) which incorporates birthweight and childhood socio-economic circumstances.

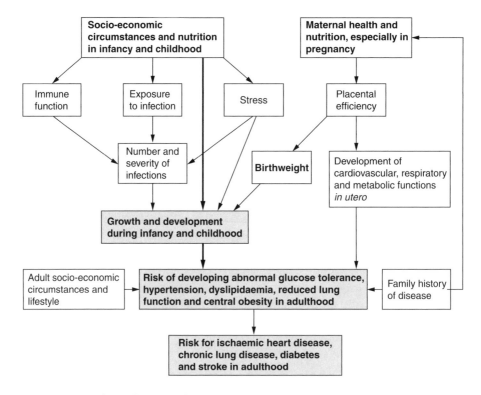

Figure 2.3: Hypothesised relationships between early life and later experience and adult disease risk (shaded boxes indicate outcome measures).

Source: Lamont *et al.*, p. 92.[67]

Although incomplete in that it does not include the impact of SES across generations and fails to link childhood SES with that in adult life, this model demonstrates plausible pathways by which fetal programming, birthweight and childhood socio-economic circumstances may combine to influence adult health outcomes. Intergenerational pathways to birthweight will be explored in the second part of this book (*see* Chapter 6).

Chapter summary

- Birthweight is a major determinant of cardiovascular mortality and morbidity in adulthood.
- The increased risk of cardiovascular mortality and morbidity is not confined to low birthweight infants but continues into the 'normal' birthweight range.
- There is evidence of a J-shaped relationship of birthweight with some adult outcomes.
- Cognitive function in early adult life appears to be associated with birthweight but weakens in later adulthood.
- Socio-economic circumstances in childhood are associated with similar adult health outcomes and there may be common pathways by which birthweight and socio-economic circumstances exert their effects.

References

1 Kuh D and Davey Smith G (1997) The life course and adult chronic disease: an historical perspective with particular reference to coronary heart disease. In: D Kuh and Y Ben-Shlomo (eds) *A Life Course Approach to Chronic Disease Epidemiology.* Oxford University Press, Oxford: pp. 15–41.

2 Barker DJ (ed) (1992) *Fetal and Infant Origins of Adult Disease.* BMJ Publications, London.

3 Barker DJ (1998) *Mothers, Babies and Disease in Later Life* (2e). Churchill Livingstone, Edinburgh.

4 Susser M and Levin B (1999) Ordeals for the fetal programming hypothesis. *BMJ.* **318**: 885–6.

5 Stafford M and Lucas A (1998) Possible association between low birth weight and later heart disease needs to be investigated further. *BMJ.* **316**: 1247–8.

6 Osmond C, Barker DJP and Winter PD (1993) Early growth and death from cardiovascular disease in women. *BMJ.* **307**: 1519–24.

7 Barker DJP, Osmond C, Simmonds SJ and Wield GA (1993) The relation of small head circumference and thinness at birth to death from cardiovascular disease. *BMJ.* **306**: 422–6.

8 Stein CE, Fall CHD and Kumaran K *et al.* (1996) Fetal growth and coronary health disease in South India. *Lancet.* **348**: 1269–73.

9 Eriksson JG, Forsén T, Tuomilehto J, Winter PD, Osmond C and Barker DJP (1999) Catch-up growth in childhood and death from coronary heart disease: longitudinal study. *BMJ.* **318**: 427–31.

10 Leon DA, Lithell HO, Vågerö D, Koupilová I, Mohsen R, Berglund L, Lithell U-B and McKeigue PM (1998) Reduced fetal growth rate and increased risk of death from ischaemic heart disease: cohort study of 15 000 Swedish men and women born 1915–29. *BMJ.* **317**: 241–5.

11 Koupilová I and Leon D (1996) Birth weight and mortality from ischaemic heart disease and stroke in Swedish men aged 50–70 years (abstract). *J Epidemiol and Community Health*. **50**: 592.

12 Martyn CN, Barker DJP and Osmond C (1996) Mothers' pelvic size, fetal growth and death from stroke in men. *Lancet*. **348**: 1264–8.

13 Rich-Edwards JW, Stampfer MJ, Manson JE, Rosner B, Hankinson SE, Colditz GA, Willett WC and Hennekens CH (1997) Birth weight and risk of cardiovascular disease in a cohort of women followed up since 1976. *BMJ*. **315**: 396–400.

14 Frankel S, Elwood P, Sweetnam P, Yarnell J and Davey Smith G (1996) Birthweight, adult risk factors and incident coronary heart disease: the Caerphilly study. *Public Health*. **110**: 139–43.

15 Whincup P, Cook D, Papacosta O and Walker M (1995) Birth weight and blood pressure: cross-sectional and longitudinal relations in childhood. *BMJ*. **311**: 773–6.

16 Forrester TE, Wilks RJ, Bennett FI, Simeon D, Osmond C, Allen M, Chung AP and Scott P (1996) Fetal growth and cardiovascular risk factors in Jamaican schoolchildren. *BMJ*. **312**: 156–60.

17 Labarthe D, Eissen M and Varas C (1991) Childhood precursors of high blood pressure and elevated cholesterol. *Ann Rev Public Health*. **12**: 519–41.

18 Gennser G, Rymark P and Isberg PE (1988) Low birth weight and the risk of high blood pressure in adulthood. *BMJ*. **296**: 1498–500.

19 Wadsworth MEJ, Cripps HA, Midwinter RE and Colley JRT (1985) Blood pressure in a national birth cohort at the age of 36 related to social and familial factors, smoking and body mass. *BMJ*. **291**: 1534–8.

20 Leon DA, Koupilová I, Lithell HO, Berglund L, Mohsen R, Vågerö D, Lithell U-B and McKigue PM (1996) Failure to realise growth potential in utero and adult obesity in relation to blood pressure in 50 year old Swedish men. *BMJ*. **312**: 401–2.

21 Law CM, de Swiet M, Osmond C *et al.* (1993) Initiation of hypertension in utero and its amplification throughout life. *BMJ*. **306**: 24–7.

22 Laor A, Stevenson DK, Shemer J, Gale R and Seidman DS (1997) Size at birth, maternal nutritional status in pregnancy and blood pressure at age 17: population based analysis. *BMJ*. **315**: 449–53.

23 Matthes JWA, Lewis PA, Davies DP and Bethel JA (1994) Relation between birth weight at term and systolic blood pressure in adolescence. *BMJ*. **308**: 1074–7.

24 Sørensen HT, Sabroe S, Rothman KJ, Gillman M, Fischer P and Sørensen TIA (1997) Relation between weight and length at birth and body mass index in young adulthood: cohort study. *BMJ*. **315**: 1137.

25 Seidman DS, Laor A, Gale R, Stevenson DK and Danon YL (1991) A longitudinal study of birth weight and being overweight in late adolescence. *Am J Diseases in Childhood*. **145**: 782–5.

26 Peckham CS, Stark O, Simonite V and Wolff OH (1983) Prevalence of obesity in British children born in 1946 and 1958. *BMJ*. **286**: 1237–42.

27 Ong KKL, Ahmed ML, Emmett PM, Preece MA, Dunger DB and the ALSPAC study team (2000) Association between postnatal catch-up growth and obesity in childhood: prospective cohort study. *BMJ*. **320**: 967–71.

28 Hales CN and Barker DJP (1992) Non-insulin dependent diabetes: thrifty phenotype hypothesis. In: DJP Barker (ed) *Fetal and Infant Origins of Adult Disease.* BMJ Publications, London: pp. 258–72.

29 Law CM, Barker DJP, Osmond C, Fall CHD and Simmonds SJ (1992) Early growth and abdominal fatness in adult life. In: DJP Barker (ed) *Fetal and Infant Origins of Adult Disease.* BMJ Publications, London: pp. 291–6.

30 Hales CN, Barker DJP, Clark PMS, Cox LJ, Fall CHD, Osmond C and Winter PD (1992) Fetal and infant growth and impaired glucose tolerance at age 64. In: DJP Barker (ed) *Fetal and Infant Origins of Adult Disease.* BMJ Publications, London: pp. 241–52.

31 Phipps K, Barker DJP, Hales CN, Fall CHD, Osmond C and Clark PMS (1993) Fetal growth and impaired glucose tolerance in men and women. *Diabetologia.* **36**: 225–8.

32 Curhan GC, Willett WC, Rimm EB and Stampfer MJ (1996) Birthweight and adult hypertension and diabetes mellitus in US men (abstract). *Am J Hypertension.* **9**: 11A.

33 Lithell HO, McKeigue PM, Berglund L, Mohsen R, Lithell U and Leon DA (1996) Relationship of size at birth to non-insulin dependent diabetes and insulin levels in men aged 50–60 years. *BMJ.* **312**: 406–10.

34 McCance DR, Pettitt DJ, Hanson RL, Jacobsson LTH, Knowler WC and Bennett PH (1994) Birth weight and non-insulin dependent diabetes: thrifty genotype, thrifty phenotype, surviving small baby genotype? *BMJ.* **308**: 942–5.

35 Wadsworth MEJ and Kuh D (1997) Childhood influences on adult health: a review of recent work from the British 1946 national birth cohort study, the MRC National Survey of Health and Development. *Paed and Perinatal Epidemiol.* **11**: 2–20.

36 Strachan DP, Griffiths JM, Anderson HR and Johnston IDA (1994) Association of intrauterine and postnatal growth with ventilatory function in early adult life. *Thorax.* **49**: 1052P.

37 Barker DJP, Godfrey KM, Fall CHD, Osmond C, Winter PD and Shaheen SO (1992) Relation of birth weight and childhood respiratory infection to adult lung function and death from chronic obstructive airways disease. In: DJP Barker (ed) *Fetal and Infant Origins of Adult Disease.* BMJ Publications, London: pp. 150–61.

38 Leon DA (1988) *Longitudinal Study: social distribution of cancer, 1971–75.* OPCS Series LS No 3. HMSO, London.

39 Ekbom A, Trichopoulos D, Adami HO *et al.* (1992) Evidence of prenatal influences on breast cancer risk. *Lancet.* **340**: 1015–8.

40 Vatten L (1996) Can prenatal factors influence future breast cancer risk? *Lancet.* **348**: 1531.

41 Depue RH, Pike MC and Henderson BE (1983) Estrogen exposure during gestation and risk of testicular cancer. *J Nat Cancer Inst.* **71**: 1151–5.

42 Brown LM, Pottern LM and Hoover RN (1986) Prenatal and perinatal risk factors for testicular cancer. *Cancer Research.* **46**: 4812–6.

43 Akre O, Ekbom A and Hsieh CC (1996) Testicular nonseminoma and seminoma in relation to perinatal characteristics. *J Nat Cancer Inst.* **88**: 883–9.

44 Tibblin G, Eriksson M, Cnattingius S and Ekbom A (1995) High birthweight as a predictor of prostate cancer risk. *Epidemiology.* **6**: 423–4.

45 Emanuel I (1986) Maternal health during childhood and later reproductive performance. *Annals of New York Academy of Science.* **477**: 27–39.

46 Marmot MG, Shipley MJ and Rose G (1984) Inequalities in death – specific explanations of a general pattern. *Lancet*. **i**: 1003–6.

47 Waaler HTH (1984) Height, weight and mortality: the Norwegian experience. *Acta Med Scand*. Suppl 679.

48 Barker DJP, Osmond C and Golding J (1992) Height and mortality in the counties of England and Wales. In: DJP Barker (ed) *Fetal and Infant Origins of Adult Disease*. BMJ Publications, London: pp. 86–92.

49 Seidman DS, Gale R, Stevenson DK, Laor A, Bettane PA and Danon YL (1993) Is the association between birthweight and height attainment independent of the confounding effect of ethnic and socioeconomic factors? *Israeli J Med Sci*. **29**: 772–6.

50 Power C, Manor O and Fox J (1991) *Health and Class: the early years*. Chapman & Hall, London.

51 Leger J, Levy-Marchal C, Bloch J, Pinet A, Chevenne D, Porquet D, Collin D and Czernichow P (1997) Reduced final height and indications for insulin resistance in 20 year olds born small for gestational age: regional cohort study. *BMJ*. **315**: 341–7.

52 Karlberg J and Albertsson-Wikland K (1995) Growth in full-term small for gestational age infants: from birth to final height. *Pediatric Research*. **38**: 733–9.

53 Sørensen HT, Sabroe S, Olson J, Rothman KJ, Gillman MW and Fischer P (1997) Birth weight and cognitive function in young adult life: historical cohort study. *BMJ*. **315**: 401–3.

54 Richards M, Hardy R, Kuh D and Wadsworth MEJ (2001) Birth weight and cognitive function in the British 1946 birth cohort: longitudinal population based study. *BMJ*. **322**: 199–203.

55 Martyn CN, Gale CR, Sayer AA and Fall C (1996) Growth in utero and cognitive function in adult life: follow up study of people born between 1920 and 1943. *BMJ*. **312**: 1393–6.

56 Strauss RS (2000) Adult functional outcome of those born small for gestational age: twenty six year follow-up of the 1970 British Birth Cohort. *JAMA*. **283**: 625–32.

57 Bartley M, Power C, Blane D, Davey Smith G and Shipley M (1994) Birth weight and later socioeconomic disadvantage: evidence from the 1958 British cohort study. *BMJ*. **309**: 1475–9.

58 Forsdahl A (1977) Are poor living conditions in childhood and adolescence an important risk factor for arteriosclerotic heart disease? *Br J Preventive and Soc Med*. **31**: 91–5.

59 Peck MN (1994) The importance of childhood socio-economic group for adult health. *Soc Sci and Med*. **39**: 553–62.

60 Wadsworth MEJ (1991) *The Imprint of Time: childhood, history and adult life*. Clarendon Press, Oxford: p. 133.

61 Blane D, Hart CL, Davey Smith G, Gillis CR, Hole DJ and Hawthorne VM (1996) Association of cardiovascular disease risk factors with socioeconomic position during childhood and during adulthood. *BMJ*. **313**: 1434–8.

62 Kuh D and Wadsworth MEJ (1989) Parental height: childhood environment and subsequent adult height in a national birth cohort. *Int J Epidemiol*. **18**: 663–8.

63 Power C and Parsons T (2000) Nutritional and other influences in childhood as predictors of adult obesity. *Pro Nutrition Soc*. **59**: 267–72.

64 Power C, Li L and Manor O (2000) A prospective study of limiting longstanding illness in early adulthood. *Int J Epidemiol*. **29**: 131–9.

65 Rahkonen O, Lahelma E and Huuhka M (1997) Past or present? Childhood living conditions and current socioeconomic status as determinants of adult health. *Soc Sci and Med.* **44**: 327–36.

66 Lundberg O (1993) The impact of childhood living conditions on illness and mortality in adulthood. *Soc Sci and Med.* **36**: 1047–52.

67 Lamont DW, Parker L, Cohen MA, White M, Bennett SMA, Unwin NC, Craft AW and Alberti KGMM (1998) Early life and later determinants of adult disease: a 50 year follow up study of the Newcastle Thousand Families cohort. *Public Health.* **112**: 85–93.

68 Spence JC, Walton WS, Miller FJW and Court SDM (1954) *A Thousand Families in Newcastle upon Tyne.* Oxford University Press, Oxford.

CHAPTER 3

The public health importance of birthweight

This final chapter of Part 1 draws together the evidence from the first two chapters that considered the impact of birthweight on child and adult health to make a case for the public health importance of birthweight. The negative impact on a range of child (*see* Chapter 1) and adult (*see* Chapter 2) health outcomes exerted by birthweight is not confined to the extreme lower end of the distribution but can be seen well into the 'normal' birthweight range. For this reason, the discussion of the public health impact of birthweight will go beyond a narrow focus on low birthweight (< 2.5kg) or preterm birth (< 37 weeks' gestation) that has preoccupied many researchers in order to explore the whole of the birthweight distribution.

In addition to its domination by attention to low birthweight and prematurity, birthweight research tends to concern itself with the effects of birthweight on individuals and the efficacy of particular therapeutic interventions aimed at overcoming the legacy of being born too small or too early. Assessment of the public health impact, by contrast, requires a population level focus. The chapter will discuss the research approaches required to examine birthweight at a population level and review the limited research on birthweight distribution across and between populations and trends in birthweight distribution over time. While avoiding an exclusive focus on the lower end of the birthweight distribution, the financial impact on a population of caring for infants born too early and too small will be considered.

Part 3 of this book is concerned with approaches to minimising the negative impact of lower levels of birthweight on child and adult health. However, for completeness, this chapter will touch briefly on the questions that the public health importance of birthweight raises for researchers, health promoters and policy makers.

Public health impact across the life course

Birthweight is associated with a range of childhood and adult health outcomes (*see* Chapters 1 and 2). These range from infant mortality through cognitive function in childhood to coronary heart disease mortality in later life.

Being born < 1500g exposes the individual to greatly increased risk of adverse health and educational outcomes even if they survive infancy. As Chapters 1 and 2 show for many outcomes as birthweight increases the risk diminishes reaching a plateau between 3500–4500g with, for some outcomes, a slight risk upturn above 4500g. In terms of risk across the life course, the optimal birthweight range appears to be between 3500–4500g. For optimum population health, as many babies as possible should be born within this optimal range and as few as possible at the high risk extremes.[1] Despite the determinist implications of the 'fetal programming' hypothesis,[2] the risk associated with birthweight appears to be modifiable by socio-economic and other factors in infancy[3] and over the life course.[4] However, consistent with the impact of birthweight observed in different populations (*see* Chapters 1 and 2), it is reasonable to assume that birthweight within the optimal range confers some protection on the individual and, within a population, the higher the proportion born within this range the better the health status of the population. As discussed below, there is some empirical evidence to support this assumption.

As far as I am aware there has been no attempt to calculate the financial burden on a society of the health effects across the life course of its birthweight distribution. However, calculations have been made of the financial burden of the health care for very low birthweight infants. Based on 1987 prices, Rogowski[5] calculated that average treatment costs per first-year survivor for Californian infants < 1500g were $93 800. Costs were graded according to the birthweight group below 1500g: $273 900 ˆor infants < 750g; $138 800 for infants 750–999g; $75 100 for infants 1000–1249g; $58 000 for infants 1250–1499g. The author points out that the cost-effectiveness of interventions to reduce the incidence of birth in these low birthweight groups would be great. For example, a shift of 250g at birth would save an average of $12–16 000 per infant in first year medical costs. Another study estimated that the initial hospital charges for surviving infants weighing 500–600g at birth averaged $1 million.[6] Much of this cost is spent on life-support equipment and many of the infants on whom large sums are spent die after as long as 100 days in intensive care.[7] None of these studies take account of the long-term costs associated with disability and educational impairment that affect a high percentage of these infants nor do they consider the financial and emotional burdens on the families.

Public health impact of birthweight

- In terms of risk across the life course, the optimal birthweight range appears to be 3500–4500g.
- For optimum population health, as many babies as possible should be born within this range and as few as possible at the extremes.
- The financial costs to a society of salvaging infants born too early or too small are very high – estimates do not include the financial and emotional burden on families or the costs of adverse health outcomes beyond the first year of life.

Birthweight measures at a population level

With the decline in infant mortality rates in developed countries and the recognition of the role of birthweight across the life course, birthweight is becoming one of the most important measures of the health status of a population.[1] This is partly because it is a predictor of mortality and morbidity across the life course but also, as will be explored in Part 2 of this book, it reflects population nutritional status and growth rates.

The birthweight of a population can be presented in a variety of ways each of which could lead to a different interpretation. The measure most often used in international statistical series and comparisons, such as UNICEF's annual report on the state of the world's children,[8] is the low birthweight rate (percentage of live births < 2500g). For the reasons discussed above, although identifying the proportion of births in the most vulnerable birthweight group, the low birthweight rate does not accurately reflect what is happening across the birthweight distribution and may fail to record important changes taking place elsewhere in the birthweight distribution.[9,10] Population mean or median birthweight (50th percentile of the normal distribution), although reflecting more accurately the birthweight of the whole population, also gives limited information about the whole distribution. This limitation is partially overcome by presentation of 10th and 90th percentiles in addition to the median and/or displaying the normal distribution curves graphically. Grouping birthweight into 500g groups (or other sub-divisions of the whole distribution) is an alternative that gives maximum information related to different parts of the birthweight distribution.[9,10] This is especially useful in view of the relationship between risk of adverse outcome and birthweight discussed in Chapters 1 and 2.

Gender and gestational age are powerful determinants of birthweight and, in order to control for these in population studies, a birthweight standard deviation score (BWSDS) has been used.[11,12] Mean BWSDS can be used to compare populations or population sub-groups; however, although this enables differences in gestational age to be controlled, it still has the same problems as mean or median birthweight in relation to the whole birthweight distribution. As with mean or median birthweight, this could be partially overcome by presenting 10th and 90th percentiles of the BWSDS. Another method which seeks to account for the number of preterm births in a population is that suggested by Wilcox and Russell[13] who have argued that birthweight distribution is not a single distribution but a 'normal' distribution with a secondary distribution of births with a pathologically low weight which can be separated mathematically from the main distribution. The secondary or residual distribution mainly consists of preterm births. For example, in a study of trends in low birthweight in Norway from 1967–1995,[14] the authors used this method to examine birthweight distribution in consecutive four-year periods. They were able to show that the increase in the low birthweight rate from 1979 to 1995, despite an overall increase in mean birthweight from 3456g to 3518g, was due to an increase in low birthweight infants in the residual distribution associated with a changed obstetric practice and assisted fertilisation. However, the method did not explain the paradox of the higher perinatal mortality rate in the Faroes compared with Denmark despite the higher birthweight in the Faroes.[15]

From the above, it is clear that population measures of birthweight need to be carefully considered and a single method may not be universally applicable or appropriate. Whichever method is chosen, it seems important to consider the whole of the birthweight distribution rather than just the lower extreme and to distinguish between the 'normal' and 'residual' distributions.

Birthweight measures at a population level

- Low birthweight (< 2500g) is the most commonly used population level birthweight measure.
- Mean or median birthweight with percentiles give more information about the whole birthweight distribution.
- Birthweight by 500g groups gives most information about the whole distribution.
- The concept, developed by Wilcox and Russell, of a 'normal' (Gaussian) distribution and a secondary or residual distribution at the left tail gives added insight into the distribution and assists comparisons between populations.

Trends in birthweight

Secular trends in birthweight have been reported to be small compared with those for height.[16] An increase of 200g over the 120 years, 1860–1984, has been reported in a study based on three Norwegian cities.[17] From the records of a US university medical centre, no significant change in the mean birthweight of term infants was noted between 1935 and 1985 but there was an increase in the proportion of infants weighing > 4000g in the final 15 years of the 50-year period.[18] Data from British national cohorts (1958, 1970 and 1986) show an inconsistent pattern (Table 3.1).[1]

Table 3.1: Birthweight trends between 1958 and 1970 in the British national birth cohorts

Birthweight percentile	1958 (National Child Development Study) (g)	1970 (Child Health and Education Study) (g)	1986 (OPCS) (g)
50th (Median)	3306	3317	3347
10th	2690	2665	2684
90th	3965	3960	3975
Mean	3315	3302	3318

Source: Alberman, p. 259.[1]

Despite a steady increase in the median weights across the three studies, the other parameters fail to show a consistent increase. Between 1983 and 1989, the percentage of livebirths $\geq$ 3500g increased steadily from 35.9% to 38.6%.[1] Using Scottish data between 1975 and 1992, Power[9] shows a similar trend to an increasing proportion of births in the birthweight groups 3500–3999g and $\geq$ 4000g occurring alongside a decreasing proportion of births in the groups 2500–2999g and 3000–3499g. Although there was no overall change in the proportion of births < 2500g, there was an increase in the proportion born $\leq$ 1500g. Similar trends were reported for the city of Sheffield for the period 1985–1994.[10] There was a small but significant increase in the mean birthweight of 34g during this period.

A shift toward bigger babies was also noted among Illinois, USA births between 1950 and 1990.[19] These authors also reported transgenerational trends: mean birthweight increases ranged from 33g for black males compared with their fathers to 74g for white females compared with their mothers. They also noted differing trends in the secondary or residual distribution with a decrease in births < 1500g among white infants by 6% compared with an increase by 56% in black infants.

Other studies from a range of countries have reported recent trends to increasing mean birthweight: Scotland 1980–92 (56g increase);[20] Austria

1970–95 (60g increase);[21] Denmark 1990–99 (45g increase);[22] Norway 1967–95 (62g increase).[14] A secular trend has also been noted in Papua New Guinea of 202g over the period 1977–1994.[23] Although an overall increase in mean birthweight was noted in the Czech Republic between 1989 and 1996 (3323g to 3353g), between 1989 and 1991 there was a sharp fall in mean birthweight of 31g.[24] Mean birthweight in ten French regions showed a different pattern: from 3290g in 1972, the mean increased to 3318g in 1981 and fell back to 3291g in 1988–89.[25] Despite significant increases in maternal height and nutritional status between two Hong Kong birth cohorts 1985–86 and 1995–96, no significant increase in mean birthweight was noted.[26]

Studies that have focused on trends in the lower end of the birthweight distribution or preterm birth rates show some contradictory trends. Reporting changes in perinatal outcomes in Western Australia between 1968 and 1976, Stanley and Hobbs[27] report a shift in birthweight distribution towards heavier babies with a fall in the proportion of infants born < 2500g from 6% to 5.3%. A study from the French region of Haguenau[28] reports a 20% decrease in the rate of small for gestational age (SGA) infants between 1971 and 1985. Live and stillbirths less than 2500g in Scotland declined slightly between 1970 and 1978 from 6.9% to 6.7%[29] and there was a significant downward trend in the live low birthweight rate in Quebec in the years 1987–1994.[30]

A decrease in the low birthweight rate from 4.2% in 1970–79 to 3.8% in 1980–89 was reported from Norway by Meberg and Broch[31] but Daltveit *et al.*[14] report a decline in low birthweight between 1967 and 1979 and a steady increase back up to the 1967 level by 1992. As discussed above, the authors attribute this increase to obstetric procedures that affect gestational age and assisted fertilisation. This is consistent with the recent report of an international study[32] suggesting that the increase in multiple pregnancies, particularly twin pregnancies, as a result of assisted fertilisation are having a major impact on trends in perinatal health indicators. A reported increase in low birthweight over a 15-year period (1978–1994) in a Brazilian study was also attributed to obstetric practices associated with elective Caesarean section.[33] An increase in the low birthweight rate from 4.97% in 1988 to 5.48% in 1995 was also reported from the Central West Region of Ontario.[34] However, Joseph and Kramer,[30] reporting on the lack of change in the proportions of low birthweight live births in the whole of Canada, suggest that the upward trend in Ontario may be due to data errors.

Two studies covering the periods from the mid-1960s through to the end of the 1980s report a trend towards decreasing rates of preterm births. A comparison of two Finnish birth cohorts 20 years apart (1966 and 1985–86) showed that overall incidence of preterm deliveries fell from 9.1% to 4.8% with a reduction from 8.8% to 3.4% in spontaneous preterm deliveries but an increase from 0.3% to 1.4% in induced deliveries.[35] The rate of preterm births decreased from 7.9% in 1972 to 5.8% in 1981 and 4.0% in 1988–89 in ten French regions.[25] The authors suggest that the improved accuracy of gestational age determination associated with the general use of ultrasound is unlikely to explain the change.

Trends in birthweight

- There has been an upward secular trend in birthweight over the last 100 years although it is less marked than that associated with height.
- Recent trends in many countries show an increase in mean birthweight of 50–60g although the pattern is inconsistent.
- Decreases at the lower extreme of the distribution have been noted but other populations have been reported to show some increase – these differences may be connected to changes in obstetric practice and the increased use of assisted fertilisation.
- There are limited data on changing preterm birth rates over time – studies from France and Finland suggest some decline in rates although these may also be modified by changing obstetric practice.

International comparisons of birthweight distribution and trends

There are major differences between birthweight distributions in different countries (*see* Table 3.2).[36]

Table 3.2: Birthweight distribution in different countries (1982–83)

Country (1982–83)	3rd centile	5th centile	10th centile	50th centile	< 1500g (%)	< 2000g (%)	< 2500g (%)	< 3500g (%)
USA – black	1651g	2043g	2416g	3186g	2.50	4.6	11.6	74
Japan	2301g	2493g	2670g	3191g	0.56	1.3	5.1	78
England & Wales	2188g	2411g	2667g	3334g	0.84	1.9	6.1	63
Denmark	2242g	2498g	2750g	3445g	0.80	1.8	5.0	54
USA – white	2276g	2498g	2750g	3447g	0.85	1.7	4.7	54
Sweden	2386g	2601g	2850g	3523g	0.64	1.4	3.7	48
Norway	2396g	2613g	2865g	3544g	0.71	1.4	3.6	46

Source: Evans and Alberman, p. 15.[36]

Norwegian infants show the distribution that is most optimal for survival and health in infancy and across the life course. Black Americans have the least advantageous distribution across the whole birthweight distribution with a very high proportion of infants in the residual or secondary distribution with birthweights < 1500g. The birthweight distribution in Japan is anomalous in that there are a very high proportion of infants born < 3500g but a very low proportion < 1500g (the residual distribution). The differences in distribution are further illustrated by Figure 3.1 that graphically contrasts the birthweight distributions of live and stillbirths for California blacks, Japan and Norway.

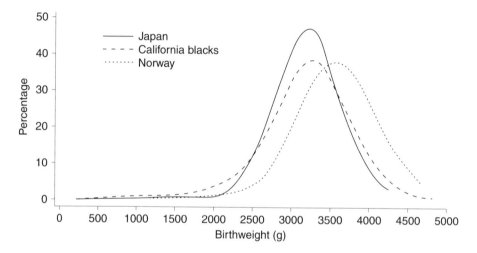

Figure 3.1: Birthweight distribution of singleton, live and stillbirths in California blacks, Japan and Norway, 1980.

Source: Evans and Alberman, p. 14.[36]

Japan has a very narrow 'normal' (Gaussian) distribution with a small residual distribution. Black Americans have a wider 'normal' distribution with a large residual distribution. Norway has a wider 'normal' distribution than Japan but shifted significantly to the right and associated with a small left tail. When trends between countries are compared (*see* Figure 3.2) it is worthy of note that the distributions in each country, although changing over time (most increasing slowly), retain the same relationship to one another.

These international comparisons confirm the importance, as discussed above, of studying the whole birthweight distribution as opposed to focusing on the lower extreme or a single measure such as the mean or the median.

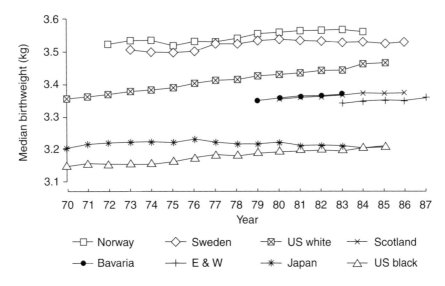

Figure 3.2: Trends in median birthweight by selected countries.

Source: Alberman, p. 259.[1]

International comparisons

- There are major differences between countries in birthweight distribution.
- Differences reflect variable proportions of births both in the 'residual' distribution and in the 'normal' (Gaussian) distribution – Japan has a low mean birthweight and a small proportion of births in the high birthweight groups but a low proportion in the residual distribution.
- Distributions in each country, although changing over time, appear to retain the same relationship to one another.

Implications for health interventions, policy and research

These issues will be more fully discussed in Part 3 but they are outlined briefly here as a logical conclusion to this chapter. The upward secular trend in birthweight that is evident in many populations is slowly affecting primarily the middle and upper ranges of the birthweight distribution. Changes at the lower extreme are variable and, especially in recent years, reflect changes in obstetric practice and the advent of assisted fertilisation. The remarkable stability of the relationship of birthweight distributions to one another over time (*see* Figure 3.2) suggests that these are either genetically determined differences or that change in birthweight may linked to intergenerational social and nutritional factors that change slowly.

Despite these constraints on rapid change, the public health impact of birthweight discussed above suggests that major health gains might accrue if health and policy interventions could be developed to reduce the residual distribution and/or shift the 'normal' distribution to the right. Joseph and Kramer[37] have suggested that potential gains in coronary heart disease mortality associated with a 100g increase in the birthweight of female and male babies would be marginal. However, because of the influence of birthweight across the life course, such an increase may have much greater effects earlier in the life course associated with later cumulative positive health effects. A marginal improvement in birthweight distribution in Scotland between 1970 and 1978 with a reduction in the proportion of births weighing < 2500g and those < 1500g was sufficient to account for 13% of the reduction in perinatal mortality between those years.[29] Saugstad demonstrates a correlation of infant mortality rates with low proportions of births < 2500g and high proportions of births > 3500g across selected developed countries (*see* Table 3.3).[38]

Table 3.3: Birthweight distributions and infant mortality rates by country (early 1970s)

Country (year)	< 2500g	2501– 3000g	3001– 3500g	3501– 4000g	> 4000g	IMR/1000
Faroes (1973)	3.7%	8.3%	26.6%	38.0%	23.4%	12.8
Iceland (1972)	4.3%	8.7%	28.2%	35.2%	23.6%	10.1
Norway (1972–74)	4.4%	11.7%	32.9%	34.3%	16.7%	10.4
Sweden (1973)	4.6%	11.9%	34.0%	33.7%	15.8%	8.6
Germany (GFR) (1973)	6.7%	14.6%	38.3%	29.7%	10.7%	21.1
Denmark (1973–74)	6.8%	17.6%	37.1%	28.5%	10.0%	10.0
Czechoslovakia (1973)	6.1%	17.1%	39.0%	28.8%	9.0%	20.4
USA (1973)	7.6%	18.2%	38.2%	27.0%	9.0%	17.7
Canada (1973)	7.0%	18.7%	39.1%	26.9%	8.3%	15.0
UK (1970)	6.8%	18.9%	39.1%	26.8%	8.3%	16.4
Poland (1974)	8.0%	19.7%	37.3%	26.7%	8.3%	23.5
Hungary (1974)	11.7%	23.4%	38.0%	21.4%	5.5%	34.3
Japan (1974)	5.1%	25.0%	46.6%	20.1%	3.2%	10.8

Source: Joseph and Kramer, p. 186.[37]

As considered above, Japan is the anomaly because of a narrow 'normal' distribution and small residual distribution. However, the relationship between higher proportions of births in the higher birthweight groups and lower infant mortality is broadly evident from these figures. The marked difference in the residual portion of the birthweight distribution between Japanese and black American infants despite the similarity in mean birthweight and the 'normal' portion of the distribution has been used to suggest that 'it is the pathological conditions that lead to an excess of small babies in the residual distribution that should stimulate public health action, not that part of the variation in birth weight which appears to be irrelevant to human health'.[39] This approach, however, fails to acknowledge the increased risk of a range of adverse outcomes (*see* Chapters 1 and 2) associated with birthweights at the lower end of the 'normal' distribution and the potential health gains associated with the shifts within the 'normal' distribution (from 2500–3499g to 3500+g) demonstrated in a number of studies.[9,10]

Further, the social differences in birthweight within populations affect the whole of the distribution not only the left tail[10,12] and, as will be discussed in detail in Parts 2 and 3, are likely to result from cumulative effects of adverse risk across time. Although genetic constraints on birthweight distribution may explain some of the differences between populations and limit the value, for example, of trying to increase the mean birthweight among Japanese infants, such constraints are unlikely to explain the differences within populations.

Rather than dismiss the potential health gains associated with upward shifts in the 'normal' portion birthweight distribution, public health interventions should be directed towards both reducing the size of the residual distribution and shifting the 'normal' distribution to the right so that more infants are born within the optimal range. A fuller discussion of these interventions can be found in Chapter 6.

Chapter summary

- Birthweight has a major impact on public health and the optimal range for most populations appears to be 3500–4500g.
- Population level measures of birthweight should include the whole birthweight distribution (means/median with percentiles or birthweight by 500g groups).
- Birthweight has a bipolar distribution – a 'normal' (Gaussian) distribution and a residual or secondary distribution at the left tail.
- There is a secular upward trend in birthweight in developed countries although less than for height.
- Trends in the last 20 years suggest increases in birthweight in many populations of 50–60g.
- Trends in low birthweight rates are less consistent.
- Birthweight distributions differ markedly between countries.

- With the notable exception of Japan, which has a narrow 'normal' (Gaussian) distribution and a small residual distribution, higher proportions of infants in the optimal range are associated with lower infant mortality.
- Public health interventions should aim both to reduce the size of the residual distribution and shift the 'normal' distribution to the right.

References

1 Alberman E (1991) Are our babies becoming bigger? *J Royal Society of Med.* **84**: 257–60.

2 Barker DJ (ed) (1992) *Fetal and Infant Origins of Adult Disease.* BMJ Publications, London.

3 McGauhey PJ, Starfield B, Alexander C and Ensmiger ME (1991) Social environment and vulnerability of low birth weight children: a social-epidemiological perspective. *Pediatrics.* **88**: 943–53.

4 Bartley M, Power C, Blane D, Davey Smith G and Shipley M (1994) Birth weight and later socioeconomic disadvantage: evidence from the 1958 British cohort study. *BMJ.* **309**: 1475–9.

5 Rogowski J (1998) Cost-effectiveness of care for very low birth weight infants. *Pediatrics.* **102**: 35–43.

6 Pomerance JJ, Pomerance LJ and Gottlieb JA (1993) Cost of caring for infants weighing 500–749g at birth. *Pediatric Research.* **4**: 231A.

7 Hack M, Horbar JD, Malloy MH *et al.* (1991) Very low birth weight outcomes of the National Institutes of Child Health neonatal network. *Pediatrics.* **87**: 587–97.

8 Bellamy C (2001) *The State of the World's Children.* Oxford University Press for UNICEF, New York.

9 Power C (1994) National trends in birth weight: implications for future adult disease. *BMJ.* **308**: 1270–1.

10 Spencer NJ, Logan S and Gill L (1999) Trends and social patterning of birthweight in Sheffield, 1985–94. *Arch Disease in Childhood.* **81**: F138–40.

11 Niklasson A, Ericson A, Fryer J, Karlsberg J, Lawrence C and Karlberg P (1991) An update of the Swedish Reference Standard for Weight, Length and Head Circumference at birth by given gestational age (1977–81). *Acta Paed Scand.* **80**: 756–62.

12 Elmén H, Höglund D, Karlberg P, Niklasson A and Nilsson W (1996) Birth weight for gestational age as a health indicator: birth weight and mortality measures at a local area level. *Eur J Public Health.* **6**: 137–41.

13 Wilcox AJ and Russell IT (1983) Birthweight and perinatal mortality: 1. On the frequency distribution of birthweight. *Int J Epidemiol.* **12**: 314–25.

14 Daltveit AK, Vollset SE, Skjaerven R and Irgens LM (1999) Impact of multiple births and elective deliveries on the trends in low birth weight in Norway, 1967–1995. *Am J Epidemiol.* **149**: 1128–33.

15 Olsen SF and Olsen J (1994) A birth weight adjusted comparison of perinatal mortality in the Faroe Islands and Denmark. *Scand J Social Med.* **22**: 219–24.

16 Cole TJ (2000) Secular trends in growth. *Proc Nutrition Soc.* **59**: 317–24.

17 Rosenberg M (1988) Birth weights in three Norwegian cities, 1860–1984: secular trends and influencing factors. *Ann Human Bio.* **15**: 275–88.

18 Johar R, Rayburn W, Weir D and Eggert L (1988) Birth weights in term infants: a 50-year perspective. *J Repro Med.* **33**: 813–6.

19 Chike-Obi U, David RJ, Coutinho R and Wu SY (1996) Birth weight has increased over a generation. *Am J Epidemiol.* **144**: 563–9.

20 Bonellie SR and Rabb GM (1997) Why are babies getting heavier? Comparison of Scottish births from 1980–1992. *BMJ.* **315**: 1205.

21 Waldhor T, Haidinger G and Vutu C (1997) Development of birth weight in Austria from 1970–1995. *Wein Klin Wochenschr.* **31**: 804–7.

22 Oskou J, Kesmodel U, Henriksen TB and Secher NJ (2001) An increasing proportion of infants weigh more than 4000 grams at birth. *Acta Obstetr Gynecol Scand.* **80**: 931–6.

23 Ulijaszek SJ (2001) Secular trend in birthweight among the Purari delta population, Papua New Guinea. *Ann Human Biol.* **28**: 246–55.

24 Koupilova I, Bobak M, Holcik J, Pikhart H and Leon DA (1998) Increasing social variation in birth outcomes in the Czech Republic after 1989. *Am J Public Health.* **88**: 1342–7.

25 Bréart G, Blondel B, Tuppin P, Grandjean H and Kaminski M (1995) Did preterm deliveries continue to decrease in France in the 1980s? *Paed and Perinatal Epidemiol.* **9**: 296–306.

26 Brieger GM, Rogers MS, Rushton AW and Mongelli M (1997) Are Hong Kong babies getting bigger? *Int J Gynecol and Obstetr.* **57**: 267–71.

27 Stanley FJ and Hobbs MS (1981) Perinatal outcomes in Western Australia, 1968 to 1976: perinatal mortality and birthweight. *Med J Aus.* **1**: 370–4.

28 Meyer L, Bouyer J, Papiernik E, Le Lann D, Moukengue L and Dreyfus J (1988) Secular trend in the rate of small for gestational age infants: Haguenau Study 1971–1985. *Br J Obstetr and Gynaecol.* **95**: 1257–63.

29 Forbes JF, Boddy FA, Pickering R and Wyllie MM (1982) Perinatal mortality in Scotland: 1970–9. *J Epidemiol and Community Health.* **36**: 282–8.

30 Joseph KS and Kramer MS (1997) Recent trends in infant mortality rates and proportions of low birth weight live births in Canada. *Can Med Assoc J.* **157**: 646–7.

31 Meberg A and Broch H (1995) A changing pattern of cerebral palsy – declining trend for incidence of cerebral palsy in the 20 year period 1970–89. *J Perinatal Med.* **23**: 395–402.

32 Blondel B, Kogan MD, Alexander GR, Dattani N, Kramer MS, Macfarlane A and Wen SW (2002) The impact of the increasing number of multiple births on the rates of preterm birth and low birthweight: an international study. *Am J Public Health.* **92**: 1323–30.

33 Silva AA, Barbieri MA, Gomes UA and Bettiol H (1998) Trends in low birth weight: a comparison of two birth cohorts separated by a 15-year interval in Ribeirao Preto, Brazil. *Bulletin WHO.* **76**: 73–84.

34 Luginaah IN, Lee KS, Abernathy TJ, Sheehan D and Webster G (1999) Trends and variations in perinatal mortality and low birthweight: the contribution of socio-economic factors. *Can J Public Health.* **90**: 377–81.

35 Olsén P, Läärä E, Rantakillio P, Järvelin M-R, Sarpola A and Hartikainen A-L (1995) Epidemiology of preterm delivery in two birth cohorts with an interval of 20 years. *Am J Epidemiol*. **142**: 1184–93.

36 Evans S and Alberman E (1989) International Collaborative Effort (ICE) on birthweight; plurality; and perinatal and infant mortality: II. Comparisons between birthweight distributions of births in member countries from 1970 to 1984. *Acta Obstetr Gynaecol Scand.* **68**: 11–17.

37 Joseph KS and Kramer MS (1997) Should we intervene to improve fetal growth? In: D Kuh and B Shlomo (eds) *A Life Course Approach to Chronic Disease Epidemiology.* Oxford Medical Publications, Oxford: pp. 277–96.

38 Saugstad LF (1981) Weight of all births and infant mortality. *J Epidemiol and Community Health.* **35**: 185–91.

39 Paneth NS (1995) The problem of low birth weight. *The Future of Children.* **5**: 20–32 (p. 25).

PART 2

The determinants of birthweight

CHAPTER 4

Biomedical determinants of birthweight

This chapter is the first in Part 2 dealing with the determinants of birthweight. The chapter deals with the biomedical determinants of birthweight including those factors associated with preterm delivery, a major contributor to low birthweight in developed countries.

As will become clear in the final chapter of Part 2 dealing with biopsychosocial pathways to birthweight, the dichotomy between biological and psychosocial determinants is misleading – as with other anthropometric characteristics such as height, birthweight is the result of the complex interaction of biological and social factors acting over time and between generations. Strict separation of these influences leads to conclusions that fail to account for complexity and necessary interaction between the biological and the social. However, to identify and characterise the components that make up the pathways considered in Chapter 6, this chapter and the next will consider determinants divided according to the convention adopted by Kramer in his methodological review of the determinants of low birthweight.[1] In this chapter, under the general heading of biomedical determinants, genetic and constitutional factors such as infant gender, ethnicity, maternal and paternal anthropometry, obstetric factors such as parity and pregnancy interval, and maternal morbidity during pregnancy including infection, pregnancy-induced hypertension (PIH) and episodic illness will be considered.

The objective of the chapter is to identify the main biomedical determinants that need to be considered in a model of biopsychosocial pathways to birthweight. No attempt has been made to carry out a systematic or methodological review of the literature but the chapter draws on a wide range of literature to achieve the objective of identifying determinants that are likely to contribute significantly to the model discussed in Chapter 6. Despite the lack of a specific methodology for including papers and weighting their quality, methodological problems in the interpretation of papers cited will be considered. Much of the literature is concerned with the determinants of low birthweight ($< 2500g$) or preterm birth (< 37 weeks' gestation) with a limited literature on the determinants of birthweight across the whole distribution. Conclusions related to the whole birthweight distribution, therefore, are necessarily extrapolated from those related to low birthweight and preterm birth.

Genetic and constitutional factors

Infant gender

Infant gender has a well-documented effect on birthweight. In developed countries, male infants have a birthweight approximately 126g higher than female infants.[1] The difference in less-developed countries is less marked – 93g.[1] Kramer[1] attributes the smaller difference in less-developed countries to the dependence of the magnitude of the gender effect on the 'ultimate potential for such growth' (p. 673). Although males have a lower risk of intrauterine growth retardation (IUGR), there is no effect of gender on gestational age.

'Race' and ethnicity

Despite being discredited as a biological and scientific concept,[2,3] 'race' remains a frequently-used predictor variable in research related to pregnancy outcomes. As a number of medical publications have now acknowledged,[3] 'race' is a social not a biological construct. The use of ethnicity as an alternative to 'race', while casting off the trappings of racist science, remains problematic as a classification. For example, the classifications most commonly used in US studies – 'black', 'white' and 'Hispanic' – are confused and confusing. Black and white refer to a biological characteristic, skin colour, whereas Hispanic refers essentially to a group characterised by the use of a common language. A similar tendency to conflate biological and cultural factors is evident in the UK classification of ethnicity.[2] A further problem is the lumping together of disparate groups into a single classification: 'Asian' in the UK classification refers to people originally from the Indian sub-continent which includes such culturally distinct groups as the Tamils of Sri Lanka and the Pashtun of the North-West Frontier; 'Hispanic' in the USA can refer to people who have been in the country for three or four generations or those who have recently migrated from Mexico or Puerto Rico; 'black' in the USA and the UK can refer to those who were born in the country or have migrated from areas of the world as different as Jamaica and Tanzania.

In response to these confusing and unscientific categories, Senior and Bhopal[4] called for improvement in the value of ethnicity as an epidemiological variable by wider recognition of its limitations, acknowledgement and avoidance of ethnocentricity, consideration of the confounding effects of socio-economic factors and recognition of the fluidity and dynamic nature of culture and ethnicity. A number of medical publications[3] have adopted these or similar guidelines. However, as will become clear in the following discussion of the evidence relating 'race'/ethnicity to pregnancy outcomes, most papers continue to treat 'race'/ethnicity as a clearly-defined variable and few adhere to Senior and Bhopal's guidelines.[4]

These methodological problems notwithstanding, there remains a body of literature documenting differences between populations (*see* Chapter 3) and sub-groups of populations (*see below*) based on these imperfect classifications of 'race'/ethnicity. These differences cannot be dismissed simply on the basis of possible misclassification of 'racial'/ethnic categories. As a potentially powerful determinant of birthweight, the literature related to 'race'/ethnicity has to be reviewed, the differences documented and explanations for these differences examined in the light of Senior and Bhopal's guidelines.[4] The place of this problematic variable in the biopsychosocial model is considered further in Chapter 6. As discussed in Chapter 3, countries have widely differing birth-weight distributions.[5] Japan's distribution is narrow around a relatively low median and a small extreme left tail (the so-called residual or secondary distribution) (*see* Chapter 3).[5] By contrast, the Scandinavian countries have a high median, a high proportion of births in the optimal range (3500–4500g) and a small extreme left tail (*see* Chapter 3).[5,6] The UK and those of European origin in the USA occupy an intermediate position and black Americans, many of whom originate from west and central Africa, have a low median and a large residual distribution (*see* Chapter 3). China appears to have a pattern similar to Japan with a low median but a small residual distribution.[1] In most countries, with the exception of China and Japan, the median birthweight and the low birthweight rate show a consistent inverse relationship such that a low median is associated with a high low birthweight rate and vice versa (*see* Table 4.1).

More recent low birthweight data show a decrease in the low birthweight rate – India in 1998/99 down to 25.5%, Pakistan in 1991 down to 21.4%, Guatemala in 1999 down to 12.4% and Hungary in 1999 down to 9.0%.[7] Mean or median birthweight data are not included for comparison with Table 4.1.

The focus of interest in research on the effect of 'race'/ethnicity on birthweight is not the differences at national level but within country differences. More specifically, it is usually ethnic minorities from less developed countries within developed countries who are the focus of interest although indigenous peoples such as Australian Aboriginals, New Zealand Maoris and Native Americans are also studied for their differences with the migrant populations of mainly European origin.

The low mean birthweight and high proportion of preterm and low birth-weight infants among black Americans has been discussed in Chapter 3. Paneth[8] reports a difference in median birthweight of 250g between black and white Americans in 1991. Among US army personnel, with according to the authors relatively equal pay and access to medical services, 3.3% of black American infants weighed less than 1500g, 7.8% from 1500–2499g, 83.2% 2500–3499g compared with 2.0%, 5.9% and 80.9% for white American infants.[9]

Table 4.1: Mean birthweight and low birthweight rate by country

Country	Mean birthweight (g)	Low birthweight rate (%)
North America		
Canada	3327	6.0
USA	3299	6.9
Europe		
France	3240–3335	5.6
Hungary	3144–3162	11.8
Italy	3445	4.2
Sweden	3490	4.0
UK	3310	7.0
Latin America		
Colombia	2912–3115	10.0
Guatemala	3050	17.9
Mexico	3019–3025	11.7
Africa		
Kenya	3143	12.8
Nigeria	2880–3117	18.0
Tunisia	3210–3376	7.3
Tanzania	2900–3151	14.4
Zaire	3163	15.9
Asia		
China	3215–3285	6.0
India	2493–2970	30.0
Indonesia	2760–3027	14.0
Japan	3200–3208	5.2
Pakistan	2770	27.0

Source: Kramer, p. 665.[1]

A study of 499 377 live singleton births in New York State in 1985–86 showed a mean birthweight difference compared with Americans of European origin of −120g for black Americans, −155g for Chinese, −235g for Japanese, −164g for Filipinos and +74g for Native Americans.[9] The risk of low birthweight was 49% higher for black Americans and 45% higher for Filipinos compared with those of European origin. The authors note that Filipinos, although classified as Asian Americans along with those of Japanese and Chinese origin, have a birthweight distribution closer to that of black Americans. Other studies have shown the higher risk of low birthweight, small for gestational (SGA) age and preterm birth among black Americans,[10–12] the similarity of Filipinos to the black American pattern[13] and the higher birthweights among Native Americans.[14]

The distribution of different ethnic groups in industrial European countries is quite different from the USA and varies according to the past colonial possessions of the country and legal and other constraints on migration from less developed parts of Europe and the rest of the world. The UK, as a result of its colonial connections with many parts of the world, has significant minorities of Indian sub-continental, Caribbean and African origin. Mean birthweight and low birthweight rate differs significantly across these groups as data from a study of 157 996 births (1988–91) in the North Thames region shows (*see* Table 4.2).[15]

Table 4.2: Mean birthweight and low birthweight rates among different ethnic groups in the North Thames region of England, 1988–91

Ethnic group	Mean (SD) birthweight (g)	Low birthweight rate (%)
White (n = 115 262)	3377 (548)	5.0
Mediterranean (n = 2642)	3299 (547)	5.8
Other (n = 2666)	3274 (567)	6.6
Oriental (n = 2351)	3231 (532)	6.6
African (n = 3905)	3214 (617)	9.2
Afro-Caribbean (n = 4570)	3156 (604)	9.4
Indo-Pakistani (n = 22 206)	3082 (527)	10.1

Source: Steer *et al.*, p. 490.[15]

The table demonstrates both the variation in mean birthweight and low birthweight rate by ethnic group and the problems associated with ethnic group classification. 'Mediterranean' is not an official classification in the UK, these groups usually being lumped together into the 'white' category. 'Other' is not specified and in many studies no distinction is made between Africans and Afro-Caribbeans, lumping them together into the 'black' category. Ethnic differences in mean birthweight at term among 10 910 deliveries based on the population of the London Borough of Croydon showed a similar pattern with the highest mean for infants of European origin (3436g) and the lowest for infants of Indian sub-continental origin.[16] The tendency to higher rates of low birthweight[17,18] and preterm birth[19] among Indian sub-continental infants and preterm birth among Afro-Caribbean infants[19] has been confirmed in other UK studies. Dhawan[20] reported an increase in mean birthweight among second generation Indian sub-continental infants in the northern English town of Bolton; however, other researchers based in Leicester reported a slight reduction.[21]

A French study based on births in a specialist unit in Paris between 1963 and 1969 reported that infants of mothers born in the Antilles had a mean birthweight (3149g) significantly lower than those infants with mothers born in France (3280g), North Africa (3277g) and southern Europe (3302g).[22] Infants born to mothers from the Antilles also had a high low birthweight rate (10%). By contrast, a better-designed Dutch study that adjusted birthweight differences for a range of confounding variables reported no difference between Dutch infants and those whose mothers were from the Dutch Antilles or Surinam.[23] Data from Australia show that Aboriginals have a lower median birthweight than those of European descent.[24] Compared with European origin infants, those with both parents of Aboriginal origin have the lowest median birthweight at each gestational age and those of mixed parentage lie in between (*see* Figure 4.1). The whole of the birthweight distribution for Aboriginal infants is shifted to the left compared with European infants – 7.5% are below the 3rd percentile, 18.1% below the 10th percentile and 71.3% between the 10th and the 90th compared with 3.2%, 10.1% and 76.9% for Europeans.[24]

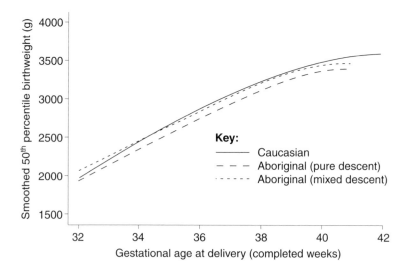

Figure 4.1: Median birthweight for gestational age: a comparison of Caucasian with Aboriginal pure-descent and Aboriginal mixed-descent infants.

Source: Blair, p. 500.[24]

A major Swedish study based on over a million births between 1978 and 1990 is interesting as it reports only minor differences in low birthweight and preterm rates between ethnic groups after adjustment for gender, year of birth, mother's age, height, parity, family type and smoking.[25] No differences compared with Swedish infants were found for infants of mothers from the Middle East, North Africa or Central and South America. Infants of Asian and Pacific Islander mothers had a slightly increased risk of preterm (adjusted OR 1.15 (95% CI 1.08,1.23)) and low birthweight (adjusted OR 1.13 (95% CI 1.04,1.22)) and infants of sub-Saharan African mothers had an increased risk (adjusted OR 1.21 (95% CI 1.05,1.29)) for low birthweight but not for preterm birth. Mean birthweights and low birthweight rates by mother's country or region of origin show some differences but not as great as would be expected from data from other developed countries (*see* Table 4.3).

Table 4.3: Mean birthweight and low birthweight rate by mother's country of origin in Sweden, 1978–90

Mother's country/region of birth (numbers)	Mean birthweight (SD) (g)	Birthweight < 2500g (%)
Sweden (1 115 906)	3513 (558)	3.6
Middle East and North Africa (21 323)	3395 (532)	3.9
Central and South America (7598)	3459 (522)	3.4
Asia and Pacific Islands (7510)	3318 (522)	5.0
Sub-Saharan Africa (2923)	3335 (566)	5.9

Source: Rasmussen, p. 447.[25]

Kramer's methodological review of literature up to 1984 led him to conclude as follows:

> although it seems clear that Blacks, Indians, and Pakistanis have lower birth weights than European and North American Whites and that certain ethnic groups (e.g. North African Jews and North American Indians) are prone to larger babies, the extent to which such ethnic differences are due to anthropometric differences, maternal nutrition, and intake of toxic substances during pregnancy has not been controlled enough to permit estimates of any independent genetic effects. (p. 675)[1]

No attempt has been made here to systematically review the literature since 1984 but it seems that the explanations for observed differences between ethnic groups remain disputed and unclear. Independent genetic effects continue to be suggested as an explanation for ethnic differences[8,26] while other studies suggest a range of clinical,[27,28] social[29] and psychological[29,30] factors that may account for the differences. Given the potential for misclassification bias resulting from the inadequate definitions of ethnicity used in many studies and the dangers of residual confounding associated with inadequately defined social status measures,[31] extreme caution should be employed before attributing independent effects to 'race'/ethnicity. However, as will be discussed further in Chapter 6, ethnicity can be fitted within a biopsychosocial model[29] to provide a better understanding of the potential relationship between constitutional and environmental factors.

Maternal height

Maternal height embodies constitutional and environmental factors reflecting genetic potential and environmental influences during the period of skeletal immaturity. Height attained is closely associated with socio-economic circumstances in childhood (*see* Chapter 2).[32] In common with other determinants of birthweight, maternal height has been studied most fully in relation to low birthweight, IUGR and preterm birth. However, there is reasonable evidence that birthweight across the distribution is positively correlated with maternal height. Table 4.4 shows the unadjusted relationship of maternal height to mean birthweight among live singleton births in Uppsala County, Sweden, in 1987.[33]

Table 4.4: Mean birthweight by maternal height in Sweden, 1987

Maternal height (cm)	Number of births	Mean birthweight (SD)
< 155	110	3264 (530)
155–159	311	3351 (608)
160–164	881	3493 (551)
165–169	1109	3566 (550)
170–174	782	3631 (534)
> 174	258	3778 (556)

Source: Nordström and Cnattingius, p. 57.[33]

Verkerk *et al.*,[23] based on 2092 births in Holland between 1988 and 1989, report a significant gradient in birthweight ratio (observed birthweight to expected mean birthweight corrected for gestational age, sex and parity) by maternal height group (< 160cm; 160–9cm; 170–9cm; > 180cm) after adjustment for ethnicity, smoking, social class, alcohol consumption, working in pregnancy and maternal age. A hospital-based study from Thailand[34] reported a similar relationship of mean birthweight to maternal height group to that seen in Table 4.4 although the mean birthweights for each group were lower. Mean birthweight for women ⩽ 150cm was 3003 (SD 446) rising steadily through the height groups to 3259 (SD 399) for women ⩾ 161cm. Similar gradients were reported from studies in India,[35] Iraq[36] and Indonesia.[37] Figure 4.2, based on a study in Guatemala, shows that the proportion of low birthweight infants (⩽ 2.5kg) falls and high birthweight (⩾ 3.5kg) increases as maternal height increases.[38]

Using multiple regression modelling with birthweight as a continuous dependent variable, Rush and Cassano[39] report a regression coefficient of 15.20 for maternal height after adjustment for parity, maternal age, marital status, social class, and smoking. This suggests that, in the study population – British births in one week of 1970 – birthweight increases by 15.20g for every centimetre increase in maternal height. From data collected between 1986 and 1991 in three hospitals in the English Midlands, Wilcox *et al.*[40] report an increase of 5.66g for each centimetre increase in maternal height after adjustment for gestation, maternal weight at booking, weight gain in pregnancy, infant gender, ethnic group, parity, smoking and deprivation score of area of residence in a multiple regression model. Wilcox *et al.*'s figure is closer to the 7.8g/cm maternal

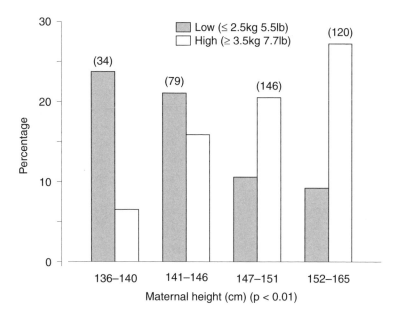

Figure 4.2: Relationship between maternal height and birthweight (number of cases given in parentheses).

Source: Lechtig, p. 554.[38]

height quoted by Kramer[1] probably because their model adjusts for maternal pre-pregnancy weight and gestational weight gain. The importance of maternal height as a determinant of mean birthweight in a population is illustrated by a study of factors influencing the increase in mean birthweight from 3326g to 3382g in Scotland between 1980 and 1992.[41] The authors conclude that changes in maternal age, parity and maternal height explain about half of the mean birthweight difference with the increase in mean maternal height over the same period from 160.0cm to 161.9cm having the largest effect. These findings are consistent with Baird's view that 'Scottish (birth) statistics are unlikely to compete realistically with those of Sweden (perinatal mortality rate of 9 per 1000) until a generation of mothers has been reared in an environment comparable to that in Sweden where in 1976 the mean height of school girls aged 16 was 65.24in (165.8cm) – at least two inches taller than in Scotland'. (pp. 1066–7)[42]

From studies of IUGR and preterm birth, maternal height is an important determinant of IUGR but not of preterm birth. Kramer[1] estimates that in a developed country with a mean height of 162cm, the population attributable risk (PAR) of IUGR associated with a maternal height of < 157.5–158cm is 6.3%. For a developing country with a mean height of 156cm, the estimated PAR is 14.5% and 18.5% for a developing country with a mean height of 152cm.

Subsequent studies in developed and less developed countries are consistent with Kramer's findings. A study based on the San Diego Prenatal Nutrition Project between 1978 and 1988 reported an odds ratio for low birthweight associated with low maternal height of 1.63 after adjustment for key confounding variables.[43] A whole population study based on the Swedish Medical Birth Register from 1992–3 reported that the risks of SGA birth increased with decreasing maternal height at all gestational ages.[44] Two studies report results for low birthweight and SGA at term: Meis *et al.*[45] show a stepwise increase in low birthweight at term with decreasing maternal height after adjustment for maternal age, maternal weight, parity, previous abortions, previous stillbirths, smoking, social class, employment during pregnancy and a range of other medical obstetric factors; Arbuckle and Sherman[46] report that only maternal height and pre-pregnancy weight remain significant independent predictors of non-preterm SGA birth after adjustment for a range of potential confounding variables.

Studies from less developed countries are fewer and at the time of Kramer's systematic review[1] there were none that fitted his methodological criteria for inclusion. A subsequently reported Indian community-based prospective cohort study showed an attributable risk for low maternal height (<145cm) of 29.5% after adjustment for low SES, maternal age, parity, short pregnancy interval, pre-pregnancy weight and low haemoglobin level.[47] Based on the study in Guatemala considered above,[38] maternal height (<145.4cm) was significantly associated with IUGR in univariate analysis but when entered into a logistic regression model along with potential confounding variables including maternal head circumference was no longer significant.[48] The authors suggest that maternal head circumference, rarely measured in studies, may be a better measure of maternal nutrition than maternal height.

Consistent with Kramer's finding[1] of no association of maternal height with preterm birth, most subsequent well-designed studies fail to show an association.[43,47–50] However, two studies show a marginal effect after adjustment for confounding variables: Meis *et al.* report an adjusted OR of 1.7 (95% CI 1.02,2.86) for preterm birth associated with maternal height <148cm with maternal height >170cm as the reference group;[51] Olsén *et al.*[52] report an OR of 1.2 (95% CI 1.0,1.5) for preterm birth associated maternal height $<10^{th}$ percentile compared with height between 10th–90th percentile. The effect sizes of these studies are too small to suggest that Kramer's conclusion is in question.

Maternal pre-pregnancy weight and pre-pregnancy body mass index

Weight, like height, is determined both by environmental and constitutional factors although, in contrast to height, it frequently undergoes change and fluctuation during adult life. Few studies relate mean birthweight to maternal pre-pregnancy weight or body mass index (BMI). Table 4.5 shows the relationship between pre-pregnancy weight and BMI based on a study in West Java, Indonesia.[37]

Table 4.5: Mean birthweight by pre-pregnancy weight and BMI in Indonesia

Pre-pregnancy weight / BMI	Mean birthweight (SD)
Pre-pregnancy weight (kg)	
< 40 (n = 83)	3013.2 (393.9)
40–< 45 (n = 132)	3098.5 (452.8)
45–< 50 (n = 125)	3063.6 (430.4)
⩾ 50 (n = 112)	3254.5 (509.5)
BMI	
< 19	3080.2 (417.2)
19–< 22	3106.8 (482.2)
22+	3192.5 (477.9)

Source: Achadi, p. 112.[37]

Despite these marked differences in mean birthweight associated with pre-pregnancy weight and BMI, neither remains significant in a multiple regression model including height, pregnancy weight gain, iron intake, illness symptoms, maternal age, parity, and various measures of socio-economic status (SES). Bhargava *et al.* present mean birthweight in maternal weight by height groups.[35] Maternal height < 145cm and weight < 45kg was associated with a mean birthweight of 2328g (SD 469) compared with 3202g (SD 489) when maternal height was ⩾ 155cm and weight > 55kg. Birthweight increased by 10.804 (SE 1.001) for each kilogram of maternal weight at booking after adjusting for a range of variables in a study from three English Midlands hospitals.[40] Data from a 1986 Finnish birth cohort[53] reported an increase in birthweight of 143.5g (SE 14.1) associated with a maternal BMI of 19.1–24.9 compared with a reference BMI of ⩽ 19 after adjustment in a multilevel multiple regression model. BMI of 25.0–29.9 was associated with an increase in birthweight of 225.0g (SE 18.3) and BMI ⩾ 30.0 with an increase of 361.8g (SE 26.9).

Kramer[1] identified pre-pregnancy weight as an important determinant of both preterm delivery and IUGR. A pre-pregnancy weight of < 54kg was associated with a relative risk of preterm birth of 1.25 and a weight of < 49.5kg with a relative risk of 1.84. As with maternal height, the PAR estimate varies with prevalence of low maternal pre-pregnancy weight. Assuming a constant relative risk, Kramer[1] estimates that in a population with a pre-pregnancy mean of 60kg the PAR for preterm birth associated with a pre-pregnancy weight < 54kg is 6.3%, for a population with a mean of 55kg the PAR is 10.3% and 14.0% for a population with a mean of 50kg. The PAR estimates for IUGR for the same population means associated with a pre-pregnancy weight of 49.5kg are 11.9%, 19.6% and 28.75% respectively. Studies published subsequently support Kramer's conclusions in relation to the effect of low pre-pregnancy weight on preterm birth[49,51,54,55] and on IUGR.[43–45,47,49] These results are consistent with the findings of a WHO collaborative study of maternal anthropometry and pregnancy outcomes based on data from 20 countries (developing and developed) that showed an unadjusted combined risk of preterm birth of 1.4 and of IUGR of 2.5 associated with maternal pre-pregnancy weight in the lowest population quartile compared with those in the highest quartile.[56]

Intergenerational and other genetic factors

The effects of maternal, and to a lesser extent, paternal birthweight and gestational age on those of their offspring have received considerable attention and have been interpreted as reflecting genetic influences on birthweight and gestational age.[26,57] Linked maternal and infant birth data from 43 891 births in Tennessee between 1979 and 1984 demonstrate a stepwise increase in mean infant birthweight with an increase in maternal birthweight (*see* Table 4.6).[58]

Table 4.6: Mean birthweight (white and black infants) by maternal birthweight group in Tennessee, 1979–84

Maternal birthweight (g)	Mean birthweight – white infants (g)	Mean birthweight – black infants (g)
≥ 4500	3635 (n = 376)	3450 (n = 62)
4000–4499	3574 (n = 1913)	3283 (n = 280)
3500–3999	3451 (n = 8323)	3250 (n = 1579)
3000–3499	3321 (n = 13 690)	3113 (n = 4101)
2500–2999	3220 (n = 6786)	3002 (n = 3354)
2000–2499	3158 (n = 1635)	2938 (n = 1065)
1500–1999	3138 (n = 288)	2943 (n = 268)
1000–1499	3127 (n = 75)	2769 (n = 64)
< 1000	3247 (n = 22)	3107 (n =10)

Source: Klebanoff and Yip, p. 288.[58]

In an earlier study in a different US cohort, Klebanoff *et al.*[59] showed a relationship of maternal birthweight to mean infant birthweight although this study suggested a J-shaped relationship with mean infant birthweight (3204g) in the lowest maternal birthweight group (2–3.9lb) higher than mean infant birthweight (3091g) in the next lowest maternal birthweight group (4–5.9lb). Based on smaller numbers (748 mother–infant pairs), Hackman *et al.*[60] reported a similar J-shaped pattern (*see* Figure 4.3). This study also showed that infants of mothers weighing ≤ 2000g were more likely to suffer unfavourable neonatal outcomes such as idiopathic respiratory distress syndrome (IRDS) and transient tachypnoea of the newborn (*see* Figure 4.3).

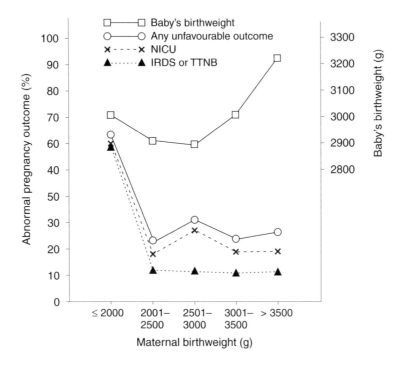

Figure 4.3: Relationship of maternal birthweight to baby's birthweight, any unfavourable outcome, need for neonatal intensive care unit (NICU) care and presence of idiopathic respiratory distress syndrome (IRDS) or transient tachypnoea of newborn (TTNB).

Source: Hackman *et al.*, p. 2017.[60]

In a multivariate regression model fitted on birthweight of the first born infants of female members of the 1958 British birth cohort, maternal birthweight for gestation was independently associated with the infant's birthweight for gestational age.[61] Each one-gram increase in maternal birthweight was associated with an 0.21g increase in infant birthweight independent of smoking at the end of pregnancy, gender of the infant, maternal height, maternal weight for height, maternal education and social class. Maternal birthweight for gestational age accounted for 4.4% of the variance in infant birthweight for gestational age after adjustment for other factors. A large Norwegian study[62] based on 11 092 mothers, reported similar results. A Swedish study,[63] based on 276 singleton term deliveries with both parents born in Scandinavia with birthweights above 2500g, reported an increase in infant birthweight of 19g for each 100g increase in maternal birthweight. Maternal and paternal birthweight combined only accounted for 5.6% of the variance in infant birthweight at term.

Kramer[1] tentatively estimated on the basis of Klebanoff *et al.*'s study[59] that maternal birthweight would explain 12% of IUGR in a population with a similar distribution of maternal birthweight. Subsequent studies throw little further light on this figure but they show mothers who were themselves SGA tend to have growth-retarded infants.[64-66] The Washington State Intergenerational Study of Birth Outcomes[67] has collected linked maternal and infant data on 46 000 births between 1987 and 1995. The relative risks (RR), adjusted for a range of confounding variables, for infant birthweight < 2500g and < 1500g by maternal birthweight group in four ethnic groups are shown in Table 4.7.

Table 4.7: Adjusted relative risks for infant birthweight < 2500g and < 1500g by maternal birthweight in Washington State, 1987–95

Maternal birthweight group (g)	Adjusted* RR (95% CI) for infant birthweight < 2500g	Adjusted* RR (95% CI) for infant birthweight < 1500g
Whites		
< 2500 (n = 1253)	1.98 (1.59,2.50)	2.28 (1.15,4.53)
2500–3999 (n = 20 216)	reference	reference
⩾ 4000 (n = 1681)	0.63 (0.44,0.90)	0.96 (0.39,2.38)
African-Americans		
< 2500 (n = 786)	1.39 (1.12,1.73)	1.22 (0.63,2.37)
2500–3999 (n = 6062)	reference	reference
⩾ 4000 (n = 261)	0.60 (0.33,1.07)	0.98 (0.32,3.06)
Native Americans		
< 2500 (n = 479)	1.73 (1.18,2.54)	0.82 (0.20,3.40)
2500–3999 (n = 6732)	reference	reference
⩾ 4000 (n = 658)	0.47 (0.27,0.84)	reference**
Hispanics		
< 2500 (n = 391)	2.16 (1.49,3.14)	1.22 (0.36,4.09)
2500–3999 (n = 5907)	reference	reference
⩾ 4000 (482)	0.59 (0.32,1.09)	0.59 (0.14,2.45)

*Adjusted for maternal age, parity, marital status, Medicaid status, smoking, prenatal care.
**Based on 2 × 2 table: maternal birthweight < 2500g vs. ⩾ 2500g.
Source: Emanuel, pp. 360–1.[67]

The risk of infant birthweight < 2500g increases as maternal birthweight decreases in all ethnic groups. Among white Americans the risk of infant birthweight < 1500g is significantly higher for maternal birthweight < 2500g but not for the other ethnic groups. The study may have been underpowered to examine risk of birthweight < 1500g in other ethnic groups.

The same study looked at the association of maternal birthweight with infant preterm birth. For births < 37 weeks, relative risks, adjusted for the confounders listed in Table 4.7, suggested an increased risk associated with maternal birthweight < 2500g of 20–30% for all ethnic groups but confidence intervals included unity in all but the African-American group. Trends across maternal birthweight groups were significant for all ethnic groups apart from Native Americans. For births < 34 weeks, the pattern was different – the adjusted relative risk associated with maternal birthweight < 2500g was 2.19 (95% CI 1.41,3.39) for white Americans with a significant trend across maternal birthweight groups (p = 0.03). Adjusted relative risks for the remaining ethnic groups suggested an increased risk with maternal birthweight < 2500g but failed to reach conventional levels of statistical significance. Significant trends were noted however for Native Americans and Hispanics but not for African-Americans. Hennessy and Alberman in their study of non-preterm gestational age in the children of the 1958 British birth cohort[61] failed to find any association of maternal weight for gestational age with gestation in the offspring. Kramer[1] also failed to find any evidence of an effect of maternal birthweight on infant gestational age. Klebanoff and Yip[58] also showed that infant preterm birth varied little by maternal birthweight. Fewer studies have examined the relationship between maternal and infant preterm birth. Kramer,[1] based on a single study,[68] suggests that about 3% of preterm infants may be attributable to maternal preterm birth. Based on 29 247 white women born in Utah in 1947–1957 and their 100 335 offspring also born in Utah between 1970 and 1992, Flint Porter et al.[69] report the results of a nested case-control study of 1405 mothers who were born preterm matched for age, multiple births, marital status, year of birth, parity and county of birth with 2781 mothers born at term. The risk of preterm birth was higher in preterm mothers than in term mothers (OR 1.18 (95% CI 1.02,1.37)). The risk increased as the gestational age at the mother's birth decreased (less than 30 weeks: OR 2.38 (95% CI 1.37,4.16)). However, neither Magnus et al.[62] nor Winkvist et al.[66] showed an increased risk in their studies.

The effects of paternal fetal outcomes on their children have received less research attention. Paternal birthweight exerted about half the effect on infant birthweight associated with maternal birthweight among term deliveries in a small Swedish study.[63] Among the children of British birth cohort members,[61] each one-gram increase in father's birthweight was associated with an increase of 0.12g in infant birthweight after adjustment in a regression model for smoking at the end of pregnancy, father's height at age 33, father's weight for height at 33, father's age at the infant's birth, father's educational qualifications and social class. Father's gestational age at birth had a small but significant effect on infant gestational age after adjustment for confounders. A Danish study showed a graded effect of paternal birthweight on infant birthweight such that compared with fathers weighing ⩾ 4kg at birth, those weighing 3–3.99kg had infants who were 109g lighter and those weighing < 3kg had infants 176g lighter after adjustment for maternal birthweight, maternal adult stature, smoking and SES.[70]

The interpretation of these familial trends in birthweight and gestational age remains a matter of debate and this will be addressed more fully in Chapter 7. However, it has been suggested that these trends support a major genetic component of birthweight accounting for between 38–80% of birthweight variance.[26,57] Johnston *et al.*[57] discuss the possible contribution of parental, placental and fetal genetic factors to birthweight. They cite the influence of parental glucokinase gene defects on birth size but do not give any indication of the likely prevalence of this defect in any specific population. Placental mosaicism, in which a cytogenetic abnormality is detected in the placenta but not in the fetus, has been reported in 1–2% of conceptuses and up to 20% of idiopathic small for gestational term deliveries have confined placental mosaicism. Among a subcohort of 758 singleton term births in the Avon Longitudinal Study of Parents and Children (ALSPAC), a significant association of the insulin variable number tandem repeat class III genotype with birthweight in children who did not change weight centile from birth to two years of age was noted.[71] Although there was no association of the genotype with birth size in the whole group, children homozygous for the class III allele showed a 200g increase in birthweight. Magnus *et al.*[72] suggest that 60% of birthweight variance is contributed by fetal genes and none by maternal genes. The size of the genetic contribution to birthweight has been challenged on a number of grounds. Little and Sing[73] report that the expression of fetal birthweight genes in males was significantly reduced if the mother smoked prior to conception. They conclude 'the gene × environment interaction described in this paper is evidence that genetic influences on birth weight are not necessarily the same in different environments. This study clearly demonstrates how treacherous it is to draw inferences about the causes of interindividual birth weight variability from models that do not properly consider the interaction between genetic and environmental factors' (p. 523).[73] Others have suggested that familial trends may be explained in part by shared family learning experience of unidentified microsocial factors related to pregnancy performance.[68] Ounsted *et al.*[74] postulate that mothers constrain the growth of their fetuses and that the degree of constraint they exert is set when they themselves are *in utero*. A recent study found that a mother's birthweight directly predicts survival of her offspring if she was < 2000g at birth.[75] The authors suggest that their findings provide an example of an 'adverse generational effect' in which prenatal experience affects a woman's subsequent reproductive success. In addition, the relatively small effect of paternal birthweight on infant outcomes supports the view that maternal intergenerational effects may reflect environmental transmission rather than genetic transmission.

Genetic and constitutional factors

- Male gender is associated with an increase in birthweight of 126g in developed and 93g in less developed countries.

- Data relating 'race'/ethnicity to pregnancy outcomes must be interpreted with caution as the classification of this risk factor is problematic. However, with some exceptions such as those of Chinese, Japanese and Native American origin, non-European origin ethnic groups in developed countries tend to have lower mean birthweights and higher rates of preterm birth.

- Maternal height is positively correlated with birthweight but shows no association with gestational duration.

- Maternal pre-pregnancy weight is positively correlated with both birthweight and gestational duration.

- Maternal birthweight, and to a lesser extent paternal birthweight, is positively correlated with infant birthweight and possibly with gestational duration.

- The relationship of maternal gestational age with infant gestational age is less clear.

- The contribution of genes to birthweight is disputed – it has been suggested that they are responsible for as much as 60% of birthweight variance but it remains to be proven.

Obstetric factors and birthweight

Parity

It is well established that nulliparity is associated with lower birthweight than multiparity. Table 4.8 shows unadjusted mean birthweight by parity from studies in four developing countries: Thailand;[34] Indonesia;[37] Iraq[36] and Morocco.[76]

The Iraqi study[36] suggests J-shaped relationship of mean birthweight with parity with grand multiparity 5+ associated with a decline in birthweight. The remaining three studies give inadequate information on grand multiparous births but the Moroccan study[76] suggests a linear rather than a J-shaped relationship. However, as Kramer[1] points out, the lack of adjustment for age, toxic exposures and SES in these studies make the results difficult to interpret. Kramer,[1] based on seven studies with a combined sample size of 83 501, calculated the sample-size-weighted effect as 43.3g per birth. A study of 9126 births in northern Finland in 1986[53] reported an increase of 144.3g (SE 10.5) in women with a parity of one to three compared with nulliparous

Table 4.8: Mean birthweight by parity group in different countries

Country and parity group	Mean birthweight (SD) (g)
Thailand	
0	3015 (443)
1	3134 (431)
2+	3167 (504)
Indonesia	
0	2978 (410)
1–2	3134 (464)
3+	3219 (469)
Iraq	
0	3030 (380)
1	3220 (370)
2	3310 (380)
3	3430 (380)
4	3500 (340)
5	3460 (490)
6	3380 (520)
7 or more	3380 (490)
Morocco	
0	3230 (SD not stated)
1	3426 (SD not stated)
2–4	3494 (SD not stated)
4+	3620 (SD not stated)

Sources: Tuntiseranne *et al.*, p. 626;[34] Achadi *et al.*, p. 113;[37] Ramankutty *et al.*, p. 7;[36] Boutaleb *et al.*, p. 68.[76]

women and 212.9g (SE 19.9) in women with a parity ≥ 4 after adjustment for confounders in a multiple regression model. Wilcox *et al.*[40] estimated that nulliparity was associated with a decrease in birthweight of 158.3g, parity one a decrease of 19.9g, parity two an increase of 29.5g and parity three and four plus with increases of 49.5g and 99.2g respectively in a multiple regression model including important confounding variables.

Kramer[1] estimates that the PAR of IUGR associated with nulliparity in a population in which half the births are to nulliparous women (most developed countries) is 10.3% and 7.1% in a population with a third of births to nulliparous women (most developing countries). Subsequent studies confirm the association of nulliparity with small for gestational age[43] and low birthweight.[46,47,49] Kramer[1] was unable to find any convincing evidence of a clinically-significant effect of parity on preterm birth. Two subsequent well-designed studies show a small effect on preterm labour[49] and indicated[77] and spontaneous preterm birth.[52,77] A study from the Ukraine[50] failed to show any effect of parity on spontaneous preterm birth after adjustment in a logistic regression model.

Birth or pregnancy interval

The effect of birth or pregnancy interval on birthweight across the distribution is not documented. However, its effect on IUGR and low birthweight has been studied. As Kramer[1] indicates, the use of birth interval rather than pregnancy interval presents a major methodological problem as, unless account is taken of gestational age, 'it is impossible to separate the effect of birth interval from the tendency for short pregnancy duration to produce short birth intervals' (p. 686). Kramer[1] reported conflicting evidence of the effect of short pregnancy interval on intrauterine growth. Most studies indicated no effect but one large US study[78] found higher rates of low birthweight associated with pregnancy intervals of less than six months. Subsequent studies show a similarly conflicting picture. A Brazilian study recorded a risk of low birthweight, adjusted for age, education, smoking and prior adverse pregnancy outcome, of 1.38 (95% CI 1.02,1.86) associated with a pregnancy interval of less than six months.[79] A US study of low-risk women in Georgia reported an increased risk of low birthweight associated with short pregnancy intervals in white and black women after accounting for potential confounders.[80] Other studies from developed[81] and developing countries[37,48,82] fail to show any effect after adjustment for confounders. However, the effect on intrauterine growth, even if demonstrated beyond doubt, is likely to be associated with a very small PAR even in populations with relatively high prevalence of short pregnancy intervals.[1,80]

At the time of Kramer's methodological review,[1] the effect of pregnancy interval on preterm birth had not been adequately studied. A study,[81] based on 10 187 women who had at least two live births in Denmark between 1980 and 1992, reported odds for preterm birth for pregnancy intervals up to 4 months of 3.60 (95% CI 2.04,6.35) and for intervals between four and eight months of 2.28 (95% CI 1.49,3.48) after adjustment for SES, age and parity compared with intervals of 24–36 months. The 'dose-response' relationship between short pregnancy interval and preterm birth in this study supports a causal relationship. Based on 4467 Bostonions who had a previous full-term live birth, Lang et al.[83] reported an adjusted OR for preterm labour of 2.0 (95% CI 0.7,5.4) associated with a pregnancy interval of less than three months.

Prior pregnancy outcomes

Prior outcomes, including intrauterine growth and gestational duration in previous pregnancies, prior spontaneous and induced abortion and prior stillbirth, are dealt with only briefly here as, with the possible exception of previous intrauterine growth and gestational duration, their effect on birthweight is minimal.[1] Prior spontaneous abortion is associated with an increased risk of preterm birth of the order of 57% and carries a PAR of 5.4%.[1] Kramer[1] found no convincing evidence of an effect of previous induced abortion on either IUGR or gestational duration.

Previous low birthweight or IUGR births are associated with reduced birthweight in subsequent pregnancies after accounting for the confounding effects of gestational age, smoking in pregnancy, gestational weight gain, calorie intake and alcohol use.[84] Kennedy *et al.*[84] estimated a birthweight decrease of 138.6g among women with a previous low birthweight infant. Rush *et al.*[85] reported a decrease of 112.8g for each previous low birthweight birth in a study in Harlem. A study from northern Finland[53] reports a decrease in birthweight of 136.2g and 253.9g associated with one and two or more previous low birthweight infants respectively after adjustment for a range of confounding variables in a regression model. Unadjusted mean birthweight for Thai women[34] with one or more previous low birthweight infants was 2830g (SD 534) compared with 3152g (SD 441) for multiparous women with no previous low birthweight infants.

Previous low birthweight or IUGR has no independent effect on gestational duration in subsequent pregnancies.[52] Previous preterm birth carries a three times increased risk of prematurity in subsequent pregnancies with a PAR of 4.9% in a population with a prevalence of prior preterm birth among multiparae of 5% and a proportion of multiparae giving birth of 50%.[1]

Obstetric factors

- Nulliparity is associated with a reduction in birthweight of the order of 100–150g and birthweight tends to increase with each subsequent birth up to parity five to six. The association of parity with preterm birth is less clear.

- Short birth/pregnancy interval is not unequivocally associated with either birthweight or preterm birth and if there is a real effect it is likely to have a small PAR.

- Previous low birthweight birth and IUGR are associated with reduced birthweight in subsequent pregnancies but not with preterm birth.

- Previous preterm birth carries an increased risk of preterm birth in subsequent pregnancies.

Maternal morbidity in pregnancy and episodic illness

Infection

There has been increasing interest in the association of maternal infection with adverse pregnancy outcomes[86] with some authors suggesting that genital tract infection may be responsible for as much as one third of spontaneous preterm births.[87] Evidence for the relationship of infections, with the exception of malaria, with birthweight is more tenuous. Kramer *et al.*,[88] in a recent assessment of the reasons for socio-economic disparities in pregnancy outcome, report that in developed countries infection has no significant aetiological role in IUGR. However, in a study of birthweight determinants among 1291 births to Aboriginal women in western Australia,[24] genital tract infection (unspecified) and recurrent urinary tract infection were associated with decreases in birthweight of 101g (95% CI 26,176) and 175g (95% CI 45,305) respectively. In a comparison group of European origin births, neither infection had a significant effect on birthweight. The failure to find an association of urinary tract infection with birthweight among European origin women is consistent with the findings from the Cardiff Birth Survey[46] showing an adjusted odds ratio for low birthweight associated with bacteriuria in pregnancy of 0.84 (95% CI 0.63,1.11).

Plasmodium falciparum malaria contributes to slowing of fetal growth and a decrease in birthweight.[1,89,90] Placental infection with falciparum malaria was associated with a reduction of 130g in mean birthweight in a study from a malaria endemic region of Papua New Guinea.[89] This effect was particularly marked in primigravidae. This finding is consistent with the deficit in birthweight (147g) with maternal malaria reported by MacGregor and Avery[91] from a study in 1969–71 in the Solomon Islands. A study from the Gambia[92] reported a 170g decrease in birthweight associated with a population rate of placental infection of 20.2%. Falciparum placental infection was independently associated with IUGR-low birthweight and preterm low birthweight after adjustment for confounding variables among women in rural Malawi.[90] The study from Papua New Guinea[89] also suggests a possible link with preterm birth. Modest support for the role of placental malaria in fetal growth retardation comes from a systematic review of interventions to prevent malaria during pregnancy in endemic areas.[93] The review suggests that chemoprophylaxis is associated with fewer episodes of fever and maternal illness and higher birthweight particularly among primigravidae.

Genital infection appears to be a determinant of preterm birth, especially birth before 32 weeks,[94] but the extent of its effect is disputed. Kramer in his 1987 methodological review[1] suggested that 'the evidence linking genital infection to intrauterine growth or gestational duration is not compelling'. (p. 708) This view is supported by a meta-analysis published in 1993 (the exact period covered by the review is not stated in the paper).[95] The authors conclude 'weak associations between infection and preterm delivery along with frequent colonization imply that infection, if involved at all, is but one of many aetiological factors'. (p. 81) However, based on subsequently reported studies, notably Hillier et al.[96] and Martius,[94] Kramer and his co-workers[88] attribute the largest portion of their preterm pie diagram (p. 199) to GU infection. Divers and Lilford[95] report the combined odds ratios separately for cohort and case-control studies for genital infection with each specific organism. They conclude that there is evidence of a weak association of *Chlamydia trachomatis* infection, *Mycoplasma hominis* (cohort studies only), and *Gardnerella vaginalis* with preterm labour and delivery but no association with group B streptococcus or *Ureaplasma urealyticum*. The meta-analysis is weakened by lack of a clearly stated search strategy and analysis of heterogeneity. The studies on which Kramer et al.[88] base their estimate of the effect of genital infection on preterm birth are large multi-centre cohort studies (10 397 in Hillier et al.'s study[96] and 106 345 in Martius et al.[94]) and a range of confounding variables are accounted for in the analyses. Hillier et al.[96] report an adjusted OR for preterm low birthweight of 1.4 (95% CI 1.1,1.8) associated with genital infection. *Vaginal bacteroides* and *Mycoplasma hominis* carry the highest risk in their study. In the 1994 Bavarian statewide perinatal survey,[94] chorioamnionitis is reported to be associated with a risk of 22.3 (95% CI 17.4,28.7) for preterm birth before 32 weeks' gestation.

Randomised controlled trials comparing antibiotic treatment with placebo or no treatment in pregnant women with bacterial vaginosis fail to resolve the question of the strength of the effect of genital infection on preterm birth. A systematic review as part of the Cochrane Collaboration[97] concludes that, despite the effectiveness of antibiotic therapy in eradicating bacterial vaginosis in pregnancy, the effect on the incidence of preterm birth (< 37 weeks' gestation) is marginal (OR 0.78 (95% CI 0.60,1.02)). The beneficial effect of treatment was most marked among women who had had a previous preterm birth (OR 0.37 (95% CI 0.23,0.60)).

Indirect support for the role of genital infection in preterm birth comes from studies demonstrating different prevalence in populations or population subgroups. Studies[27,98,99] among different ethnic groups in the USA show a higher prevalence of bacterial vaginosis among black American women in pregnancy compared with other ethnic groups. These studies suggest that the increased prevalence of vaginosis may explain some of the ethnic differences in preterm delivery. A similar difference in prevalence of genital infection in pregnancy has been noted among Aboriginal women in Australia compared with those of European origin.[24] Prevalence was also reported to be low among Hong Kong Chinese women who have a low preterm birth rate.[100]

Kramer[1] was unable to find any convincing evidence for an effect of urinary tract infection or asymptomatic bacteriuria on gestational duration. A meta-analysis of the relationship between asymptomatic bacteriuria and preterm delivery published in 1989 (two years after Kramer[1]), however, reported that non-bacteriuric women had about two-thirds lower risk (OR 0.50 (95% CI 0.36,0.70)) of preterm delivery compared with bacteriuric women.[101] Later reports suggest some association: Schieve et al.[102] based on a cohort of 25 746 report a significant association of urinary tract infection with prematurity; in the Cardiff Birth Survey,[51] bacteriuria had a marginal effect in a model with medical factors alone but not when other confounding variables were included in the model.

A Cochrane review of antibiotic treatment for asymptomatic bacteriuria in pregnancy[103] lends some weak support to the role of bacteriuria in preterm delivery. The analysis shows a significant reduction in preterm delivery associated with treatment (OR 0.60 (95% CI 0.45,0.80)) but the author cautions that the poor methodological quality of the studies means definitive conclusions for this outcome remain questionable. A further systematic review published in 1998[104] reaches a similar conclusion – treatment of asymptomatic bacteriuria reduces the incidence of preterm birth (OR 0.67 (95% CI 0.52,0.85)).

General morbidity and episodic illness

Kramer in his 1987 methodological review[1] reported that episodic illness in pregnancy may be associated with a reduction in birthweight of between 44.7g[105] and 80.8g.[106] However, he concludes 'there is little available information on the effects of episodic maternal illness on intrauterine growth, and almost none on pregnancy duration' (p. 704).[1] A subsequent well-designed Indonesian study[57] with adequate power showed no effect of maternal illness on birthweight in multiple regression model including social, anthropometric and obstetric variables. A study[107] with a sample of only 121 births in Papua New Guinea reported an association of maternal illness with preterm birth. Major studies in developed countries such as the Cardiff Birth Survey[51] and other European studies[23,52] have not studied this potential association with adverse pregnancy outcomes. Kramer et al.[88] do not include maternal episodic illness in either their IUGR or preterm pie diagrams suggesting that, at least in developed countries, based on existing evidence maternal episodic illness is not a significant determinant of adverse pregnancy outcome.

Pre-existing and PIH

Pregnancy-induced hypertension (PIH) is an important determinant of IUGR and preterm birth with a PAR of approximately 10% for each outcome.[88] Less is known about the role of pre-existing hypertension. Pre-pregnancy hypertension was independently associated with spontaneous preterm birth in a cohort of 13 102 women giving birth in Montreal between 1980 and 1989.[108] Monaghan *et al.*[50] reported an odds ratio of 2.3 (95% CI 0.9,5.2) for spontaneous preterm birth associated with pre-existing hypertension (measured before 27 weeks' gestation) after adjustment for major confounders. In a population with 4.5% spontaneous preterm births and a prevalence of 2.7% hypertension in early pregnancy (as in this study) the PAR using the formula quoted in Kramer[1] (p. 669) would be 2.7%. A history of chronic hypertension was a significant risk factor for indicated but not spontaneous preterm birth in a multi-centre US study.[109] Clinical hypertension before the 20th week of pregnancy was associated with a decrease in birthweight of 116g after adjustment for confounding in a multiple regression model among northern Finnish women.[53]

Pregnancy-induced hypertension without proteinuria decreased birthweight by 66g (SE 14.7) in the northern Finnish study[53] whereas pre-eclampsia (PIH with proteinuria) was associated with a decrease of 160.4g (SE 33.6). A prospective study[110] of 209 nulliparous women booked for antenatal care at a London hospital found that an increase in mean 24-hour diastolic blood pressure at 28 weeks' gestation was associated with a 68g (95% CI 3,132) decrease in birthweight and a similar change in diastolic pressure at 36 weeks' gestation with a 76g (95% CI 24,129) decrease independent of age, smoking, height, weight, alcohol intake, ethnic origin and gestation. Pre-eclampsia was significantly associated with lower birthweight in both the 1958 and 1970 British birth cohorts.[111]

The unadjusted risk of a SGA birth was 2.84 (95% CI 1.9,4.2) with hypertension without proteinuria in a case-control study based on births in Oxford between 1964 and 1977.[112] The risk associated with pre-eclampsia was 15.78 (95% CI 6.2,40.4). Pre-eclampsia but not essential hypertension increased the risk (adjusted OR 2.4 (95% CI 1.4,4.1)) of SGA birth among multiparae without a previous SGA birth in an Australian study.[113] Neither pre-eclampsia nor essential hypertension, however, was included in the final model among women with a previous SGA birth. PIH (adjusted OR 1.56 (1.28,1.89)) and pre-eclampsia (adjusted OR 4.80 (3.59,6.41)) were both implicated as significant risk factors for low birthweight in the Cardiff Birth Survey.[46] Other studies report an increased risk of low birthweight associated with PIH[27,114–116] and pre-eclampsia.[117,118]

Pregnancy-induced hypertension is associated with an increased risk of preterm birth in a number of studies. A large study in Montreal[108] reports an independent association of severe PIH with preterm birth as does a study of Aboriginal births in Darwin Health Region, Australia.[119] Other studies report a relationship but do not adjust for confounding variables.[116,120,121] The Cardiff

Birth Survey, however, fails to show an association with PIH without protein-uria once other confounding factors are taken into account although pre-eclampsia remains significantly related.[51]

Maternal illness and birthweight

- Malarial infection of the placenta is associated with a decrease in birthweight in the order of 150–170g.
- There is increasing evidence for an association of genital infection with preterm birth although the extent of the effect is disputed.
- The association of urinary tract infection and asymptomatic bacteriuria with preterm birth is less clear.
- The evidence for an association of maternal episodic illness with birth-weight or gestational duration is scanty.
- Pregnancy-induced hypertension appears to be associated both with reduction in birthweight and gestational duration.

The role of biomarkers

While not strictly biological risk factors for birthweight or gestational duration, biomarkers reflect the proximal biological pathways by which some of the risks discussed above exert their influence on pregnancy outcomes. This very brief review of the main markers is intended to inform subsequent discussion of the mechanisms by which biopsychosocial factors combine to influence birthweight and pregnancy duration. Chuileannain and Brennecke[122] summarise the bio-markers that may prove valuable in predicting preterm labour. Inflammatory cytokines (interleukin-1 β, tumour necrosis factor α, interleukin-6 (IL-6) and interleukin-8 (IL-8)) have been studied in relation to their role in the initiation of labour. IL-6 has been the main focus – it is thought that raised levels in amniotic fluid in the second trimester may be associated with pre-existing subclinical infection (*see above*). Elevated maternal serum IL-6 concentrations may be a predictor of preterm labour and delivery in women in threatened preterm labour with or without subclinical intrauterine infection. Disruption of the chorionic-decidual interface may precede the onset of labour and remodelling of the extracellular matrix (ECM) may lead to this disruption which in turn may permit the release of ECM components such as fetal fibronectin (fFN) into the cervicovaginal fluid. The presence of fFN in cervicovaginal fluid at concentrations of > 50ng/ml between 21 and 37 weeks' gestation is predict-ive of preterm delivery.

Unexplained increases in midtrimester maternal serum human chorionic gonadotropin (hCG) have been shown to be associated with higher prevalence of both IUGR and preterm delivery.[123–125] In combination with increased serum α-fetoprotein and low unconjugated oestriol, increased serum hCG has been shown to have the potential as a multiple screening tool in the detection of high-risk pregnancies.[124]

Recent interest in relation to preterm birth has focused on maternal plasma corticotropin-releasing hormone (CRH).[126] A number of studies[127,128] have recorded a relationship between increased CRH at various stages of pregnancy with preterm delivery. An interesting link with psychosocial factors and biological factors in the determination of preterm birth is the suggested role of stress in promoting increased secretion of CRH contributing to bio-pathways to preterm birth.[126,129] In this context, it is significant that Kramer *et al.*[130] include CRH as the main biomarker in their ongoing of pathways from low SES to preterm birth.

Multiple births: an explanation

A notable omission from this chapter is a discussion of the role of multiple pregnancies in relation to birthweight and gestational duration. I initially took a decision in thinking about this book to focus primarily on singleton births as the relationship between multiple births and low birthweight/short gestational duration was well-established and was unlikely to be affected by social or psychological factors. I did not consider it likely that multiple pregnancy would be an important component in biopsychosocial pathways to birthweight. However, a recent paper[131] suggests that, as a consequence of assisted fertilisation, multiple births, particularly twin deliveries, have a major population-based impact on the trends of perinatal health indicators. There is also some evidence that the higher use of assisted fertilisation among higher social groups may be influencing social patterning of birthweight and gestational duration through the higher incidence of low birthweight and preterm births among multiple births resulting from these procedures.

Although the omission of multiple pregnancy from the models proposed in Chapters 6 and 7 may limit their application to the changing situation brought about by advances in obstetric practice, the focus on singleton births remains valid as they continue to form the vast majority of births in all countries.

Chapter summary

- Constitutional and genetic factors such as gender, maternal height and pre-pregnancy weight, maternal birthweight and possibly gestational age are associated with increased birthweight.

- Ethnicity also seems to be associated with birthweight although, like maternal height and pre-pregnancy weight, social and environmental factors may well determine some of the differences noted between ethnic groups.

- Obstetric factors such as parity, previous low birthweight birth and previous preterm birth are associated with birthweight although only previous preterm birth has been shown to have a definite relationship with gestational duration.

- Maternal illness influences birthweight and gestational duration primarily through PIH and genital infection. In developing countries malaria significantly lowers birthweight.

- Biomarkers, although not themselves risk factors for birthweight or gestational duration, reflect the proximal biological pathways by which some of the above factors exert their influence on pregnancy outcomes. CRH is of particular interest as a biomarker for preterm birth.

References

1 Kramer MS (1987) Determinants of low birth weight: methodological assessment and meta-analysis. *Bull WHO.* **65**: 663–737.

2 Spencer NJ (1996) Race and ethnicity as determinants of child health: a personal view. *Child: Care, Health and Dev.* **22**: 327–46.

3 British Medical Journal (1996) Style matters. Ethnicity, race and culture: guidelines for research, audit and publication. *BMJ.* **312**: 1094.

4 Senior PA and Bhopal R (1994) Ethnicity as a variable in epidemiological research. *BMJ.* **309**: 327–30.

5 Alberman E (1991) Are our babies becoming bigger? *J Royal Society of Med.* **84**: 257–60.

6 Saugstad LF (1981) Weight of all births and infant mortality. *J Epidemiol and Community Health.* **35**: 185–91.

7 UNICEF (2002) End of Decade Databases: www.childinfo.org/eddb/lbw/index.htm (accessed 20.2.02).

8 Paneth NS (1995) The problem of low birth weight. *The Future of Children.* **5**: 20–32 (p. 25).

9 Singh GK and Yu SM (1994) Birth weight differentials among Asian-Americans. *Am J Public Health.* **84**: 1444–9.

10 Goldenberg RL, Cliver SP, Cutter GR, Hoffman HJ, Cassidy G, Davis RO and Nelson GK (1991) Black-white differences in newborn anthropometric measurements. *Obstetr and Gynecol.* **78**: 782–8.

11 McGrady GA, Sung JF, Rowley DL and Hogue CJ (1992) Preterm delivery and low birth weight among first-born infants of black and white college graduates. *Am J Epidemiol.* **136**: 266–76.

12 Schieve LA and Handler A (1996) Preterm delivery and perinatal death among black and white infants in a Chicago-area perinatal registry. *Obstetr and Gynecol.* **88**: 356–63.

13 Alexander GR, Baruffi G, Mor J and Kieffer E (1992) Maternal nativity status and pregnancy outcome among US-born Filipinos. *Soc Biol.* **39**: 278–84.

14 Buck GM, Mahoney MC, Michalek AM, Powell EJ and Shelton JA (1992) Comparison of Native American births in upstate New York with other race births. *Public Health Rep.* **107**: 569–75.

15 Steer P, Alam MA, Wadsworth J and Welch A (1995) Relation between maternal haemo-globin concentration and birth weight in different ethnic groups. *BMJ.* **310**: 489–91.

16 Lyon AJ, Clarkson P, Jeffrey I and West GA (1994) Effect of ethnic origin of mother on fetal outcome. *Arch Disease in Childhood.* **70**: F40–3.

17 Versi E, Liu KL, Chia P and Seddon G (1995) Obstetric outcome of Bangladeshi women in East London. *Br J Obstetr and Gynaecol.* **102**: 630–7.

18 Jivani SK (1986) Asian neonatal mortality in Blackburn. *Arch of Disease in Childhood.* **61**: 510–2.

19 Gardosi J and Francis A (2000) Early pregnancy predictors of preterm birth: the role of a prolonged menstruation-conception interval. *Br J Obstetr and Gynaecol.* **107**: 228–37.

20 Dhawan S (1995) Birth weights of infants of first generation Asian women in Britain compared with second generation Asian women. *BMJ.* **310**: 86–8.

21 Draper E, Abrams KR and Clarke M (1995) Fall in birth weight of third generation Asian infants. *BMJ.* **311**: 876.

22 Kaminski M, Goujard J and Rumeau-Rouquette C (1975) La grossesse des femmes migrantes à Paris. *Rev Français Gynécol.* **70**: 483–91.

23 Verkerk PH, Zaadstra JD, Reerink JD, Herngreen WP and Verloove-Vanhorick SP (1994) Social class, ethnicity and other risk factors for small for gestational age and preterm delivery in the Netherlands. *Eur J Obstetr and Gynecol.* **53**: 129–34.

24 Blair E (1996) Why do Aboriginal newborns weigh less? Determinants of birthweight for gestational age. *J Paed and Child Health.* **32**: 498–503.

25 Rasmussen F, Oldenburg CEM, Ericson A and Gunnarskog J (1995) Preterm birth and low birthweight among children of Swedish and immigrant women between 1978 and 1990. *Paed and Perinatal Epidemiol.* **9**: 441–54.

26 Hoffman J and Ward K (1999) Genetic factors in preterm delivery. *Obstetr and Gynecol Survey.* **54**: 203–10.

27 Kempe A, Wise PH, Barkan SE, Sappenfield WM, Sachs B, Gortmaker SL, Sobol AM, First LR, Pursley D, Rinehart H, Kotelchuck M, Sessions Cole F, Gunter N and Stockbauer JW (1992) Clinical determinants of the racial disparity in very low birth weight. *New England J Med.* **327**: 969–73.

28 Goldenburg RL, Klebanoff MA, Nugent R, Krohn MA, Hillier S and Andrews WW (1996) Bacterial colonization of the vagina during pregnancy in four ethnic groups. *Am J Obstetr and Gynecol.* **174**: 1618–21.

29 Reeb KG, Graham AV, Zyzanski SJ and Kitson GC (1987) Predicting low birthweight and complicated labor in urban black women: a biopsychosocial perspective. *Soc Sci and Med.* **25**: 1321–7.

30 Blackmore CA, Ferré CD, Rowley DL, Hogue CJR, Gaiter J and Atrash H (1993) Is race a risk factor or a risk marker for preterm delivery? *Ethnicity Dis.* **3**: 372–7.

31 Davey Smith G and Phillips AN (1992) Confounding in epidemiological studies: why 'independent' effects may not be what they seem. *BMJ.* **305**: 757–9.

32 Kuh D and Wadsworth MEJ (1989) Parental height: childhood environment and subsequent adult height in a national birth cohort. *Int J Epidemiol.* **18**: 663–8.

33 Nordström M-L and Cnattingius S (1996) Effects on birthweights of maternal education, socio-economic status and work-related characteristics. *Scand J Soc Med.* **24**: 55–61.

34 Tuntiseranee P, Olsen J, Chongsuvivatwong V and Limbutara S (1999) Socioeconomic and work related determinants of pregnancy outcome in southern Thailand. *J Epidemiol and Community Health.* **53**: 624–9.

35 Bhargava V, Chatterjee M, Prakash A, Bhatia B and Mishra A (1983) Fetal growth variations: I. Influence of maternal size and nutrition on identification of fetal growth retardation. *Ind Pediatrics.* **20**: 549–59.

36 Ramankutty P, Tikreeti RAS, Rasaam KW, Al-Thamery DM, Yacoub AAH and Mahmood DA (1983) A study on birth weight of Iraqi children. *J Trop Pediatr.* **29**: 5–10.

37 Achadi EL, Hansell MJ, Sloan NL and Anderson MA (1995) Women's nutritional status, iron consumption and weight gain during pregnancy in relation to neonatal weight and length in West Java, Indonesia. *Int J Gynecol and Obstetr.* **48** (Suppl): S103–19.

38 Lechtig A, Delgado H, Lasky R, Yarbrough C, Klein RE, Habicht J-P and Béhar M (1975) Maternal nutrition and fetal growth in developing societies. *Am J of Disease in Childhood.* **129**: 553–6.

39 Rush D and Cassano P (1983) Relationship of cigarette smoking and social class to birth weight and perinatal mortality among all births in Britain, 5–11 April 1970. *J Epidemiol and Community Health.* **37**: 249–55.

40 Wilcox MA, Smith SJ, Johnson IR, Maynard PV and Chilvers CED (1995) The effect of social deprivation on birthweight, excluding physiological and pathological effects. *Br J Obstetr and Gynaecol.* **102**: 918–24.

41 Bonellie SR and Raab GM (1997) Why are babies getting heavier? Comparison of Scottish births from 1980 to 1992. *BMJ.* **315**: 1205.

42 Baird D (1980) Environment and reproduction. *Br J Obstetr and Gynaecol.* **87**: 1057–67.

43 Abrams B and Newman V (1991) Small-for-gestational age birth: maternal predictors and comparison with risk factors for spontaneous preterm delivery in the same cohort. *Am J Obstetr and Gynecol.* **164**: 785–90.

44 Clausson B, Cnattingius S and Axelsson O (1998) Preterm and term births of small for gestational age infants: a population-based study of risk factors among nulliparous women. *Br J Obstetr and Gynaecol.* **105**: 1011–7.

45 Meis PJ, Michielutte R, Peters TJ, Bradley Wells H, Evan Sands R, Coles EC and Johns KA (1997) Factors associated with term low birthweight in Cardiff, Wales. *Paed and Perinatal Epidemiol.* **11**: 287–97.

46 Arbuckle TE and Sherman GJ (1989) Comparison of the risk factors for pre-term delivery and intrauterine growth retardation. *Paed and Perinatal Epidemiol.* **3**: 115–29.

47 Hirve SS and Ganatra BR (1994) Determinants of low birth weight: a community based prospective cohort study. *Ind Pediatrics.* **31**: 1221–5.

48 Villar J, Khoury MJ, Finucane FF and Delgado HL (1986) Differences in the epidemiology of prematurity and intrauterine growth retardation. *Early Human Dev.* **14**: 307–20.

49 Lang JM, Lieberman E and Cohen A (1996) A comparison of risk factors for preterm labor and term small for gestational age birth. *Epidemiol.* **7**: 369–76.

50 Monaghan SC, Little RE, Hulchiy O, Strassner H and Claden BC (2001) Risk factors for spontaneous preterm birth in two urban areas of Ukraine. *Paed and Perinatal Epidemiol.* **15**: 123–30.

51 Meis PJ, Michielutte R, Peters TJ, Bradley Wells H, Evan Sands R, Coles EC and Johns KA (1995) Factors associated with preterm birth in Cardiff, Wales: I. Univariable and multivariable analysis. *Am J Obstetr and Gynecol.* **173**: 590–6.

52 Olsén P, Läärä E, Rantakillio P, Järvelin M-R, Sarpola A and Hartikainen A-L (1995) Epidemiology of preterm delivery in two birth cohorts with an interval of 20 years. *Am J Epidemiol.* **142**: 1184–93.

53 Järvelin M-R, Elliott P, Kleinschmidt I, Martuzzi M, Grundy C, Hartikainen A-L and Rantakillio P (1997) Ecological and individual predictors of birthweight in a northern Finland birth cohort, 1986. *Paed and Perinatal Epidemiol.* **11**: 298–312.

54 Ferraz EM, Gray RH and Cunha TM (1990) Determinants of preterm delivery and intrauterine growth retardation in north-east Brazil. *Int J Epidemiol.* **19**: 101–8.

55 Lumme R, Rantakallio P, Hartikainen A-L and Järvelin M-R (1995) Pre-pregnancy weight and its relation to pregnancy outcome. *J Obstetr and Gynaecol.* **15**: 69–75.

56 WHO Collaborative Study (1995) Maternal anthropometry and pregnancy outcomes. *Bull WHO.* **73** (Suppl): 1–98.

57 Johnston LB, Clark AJL and Savage MO (2002) Genetic factors contributing to birth weight. *Arch Disease in Childhood.* **86**: Fetal and Neonatal Edition F2–3.

58 Klebanoff MA and Yip R (1987) Influence of maternal birth weight on rate of fetal growth and duration of gestation. *J Pediatrics.* **111**: 287–92.

59 Klebanoff MA, Graubard BI, Kessel SS and Berendes HW (1984) Low birth weight across generations. *JAMA.* **252**: 2423–7.

60 Hackman E, Emanuel I, van Belle G and Daling J (1983) Maternal birth weight and subsequent pregnancy outcome. *JAMA.* **250**: 2016–9.

61 Hennessy E and Alberman E (1998) Intergenerational influences affecting birth outcome: I. Birthweight for gestational age in the children of the 1958 British Birth Cohort. *Paed and Perinatal Epidemiol.* **12** (Suppl 1): 45–60.

62 Magnus P, Bakketeig LS and Skjærven R (1993) Correlations of birthweight and gestational age across generations. *Ann Human Biol.* **20**: 231–8.

63 Langhoff-Roos J, Lindmark G, Gustavson K-H, Gebre-Medhin M and Meirik O (1987) Relative effect of parental birth weight on infant birth weight at term. *Clin Genetics.* **32**: 240–8.

64 Klebanoff MA, Schulsinger C, Mednick BR and Secher NJ (1997) Preterm and small for gestational age birth across generations. *Am J Obstetr and Gynecol.* **176**: 521–6.

65 Klebanoff MA, Meirik O and Berendes HW (1989) Second generation consequences of small for dates birth. *Pediatrics.* **84**: 343–7.

66 Winkvist A, Mogren I and Hogberg U (1998) Familial patterns in birth characteristics: impact on individual and population risks. *Int J Epidemiol.* **27**: 248–54.

67 Emanuel I, Leisenring W, Williams MA, Kimpo C, Estee S, O'Brien W and Hale CB (1999) The Washington State Intergenerational Study of Birth Outcomes: methodology and some comparisons of maternal birthweight and infant birthweight and gestation in four ethnic groups. *Paed and Perinatal Epidemiol.* **13**: 352–71.

68 Johnstone F and Inglis L (1974) Familial trends in low birth weight. *BMJ.* **3**: 659–61.

69 Flint Porter T, Fraser AM, Hunter CY, Ward RH and Varner MW (1997) The risk of preterm birth across generations. *Obstetr and Gynecol.* **90**: 63–7.

70 Klebanoff MA, Mednick BR, Schulsinger C, Secher NJ and Shiono PH (1998) Father's effect on infant birth weight. *Am J Obstetr and Gynecol.* **178**: 1022–6.

71 Dunger DB, Ong KK, Huxtable SJ, Sherriff A, Woods KA, Ahmed ML, Golding J, Pembreey ME, Ring S, Bennett ST and Todd JA (1998) Association of the INS VNTR with size at birth: ALSPAC study team. *Nature Genetics.* **19**: 98–100.

72 Magnus P, Berg K, Bjerkedal T and Nance WE (1984) Parental determinants of birth weight. *Clin Genetics.* **26**: 397–405.

73 Little RE and Sing CF (1987) Genetic and environmental influences on human birth weight. *Am J Human Genetics.* **40**: 512–26.

74 Ounsted M, Scott A and Ounsted C (1986) Transmission through the female line of a mechanism constraining human fetal growth. *Ann Human Biol.* **13**: 143–51.

75 Skjærven R, Wilcox AJ, Øyen N and Magnus P (1997) Mother's birth weight and survival of their offspring: population based study. *BMJ.* **314**: 1376–80.

76 Boutaleb Y, Lahlou N, Oudghiri A and Mesbahi M (1982) Le poids de naissance dans un pays africain. *J Gynécol, Obstétr et Biol Repro.* **11**: 68–72.

77 Meis PJ, Michielutte R, Peters TJ, Bradley Wells H, Evan Sands R, Coles EC and Johns KA (1995) Factors associated with preterm birth in Cardiff, Wales: II. Indicated and spontaneous preterm birth. *Am J Obstetr and Gynecol.* **173**: 597–602.

78 Eisner V, Brazie JV, Pratt MW and Hexter AC (1979) The risk of low birthweight. *Am J Public Health.* **69**: 887–93.

79 Ferraz EM, Gray RH, Fleming PL and Maia TM (1988) Interpregnancy interval and low birth weight: findings from a case-control study. *Am J Epidemiol.* **128**: 1111–6.

80 Adams MM, Delaney KM, Stupp PW, McCarthy BJ and Rawlings JS (1997) The relationship of interpregnancy interval to infant birthweight and length of gestation among low-risk women, Georgia. *Paed and Perinatal Epidemiol.* **11** (Suppl 1): 48–62.

81 Basso O, Olsen J, Knudsen LB and Christensen K (1998) Low birth weight and preterm birth after short interpregnancy intervals. *Am J Obstetr and Gynecol.* **178**: 259–63.

82 Fourn L, Goulet L and Seguin L (1996) Pregnancy intervals and low birthweight in Benin. *Med Trop.* **56**: 163–6.

83 Lang JM, Lieberman E, Ryan KJ and Monson RR (1990) Interpregnancy interval and risk of preterm labor. *Am J Epidemiol.* **132**: 304–9.

84 Kennedy ET, Gershoff S, Reed R and Austin JE (1982) Evaluation of the effect of WIC supplemental feeding on birth weight. *J Am Dietetic Assoc.* **80**: 220–7.

85 Rush D, Davis H and Susser M (1972) Antecedents of low birthweight in Harlem, New York. *Int J Epidemiol.* **1**: 375–87.

86 Brocklehurst P (1999) Infection and preterm labour. *BMJ.* **318**: 548–9.

87 McDonald HM, O'Loughlin JA, Vigneswaran R, Jolley PT, Harvey JA, Bof A and McDonald PJ (1997) Impact of metronidazole on preterm birth in women with bacterial vaginosis flora (*Gardnerella vaginalis*): a randomised, placebo controlled trial. *Br J Obstetr and Gynaecol.* **104**: 1391–7.

88 Kramer MS, Séguin L, Lydon J and Goulet L (2000) Socio-economic disparities in pregnancy outcome: why do the poor fare so poorly? *Paed and Perinatal Epidemiol.* **14**: 194–210.

89 Allen SJ, Raiko A, O'Donnell A, Alexander NDE and Clegg JB (1998) Causes of preterm delivery and intrauterine growth retardation in a malaria endemic region of Papua New Guinea. *Arch Disease in Childhood.* **79**: Fetal and Neonatal Edition F135–40.

90 Steketee RW, Wirima JJ, Hightower AW, Slutsker L, Heymann DL and Breman JG (1996) The effect of malaria and malaria prevention in pregnancy on offspring birthweight, prematurity and intrauterine growth retardation in rural Malawi. *Am J Trop Med and Hygiene.* **55** (Suppl 1): 33–41.

91 MacGregor JD and Avery JG (1974) Malaria transmission and fetal growth. *BMJ.* **3**: 433–6.

92 MacGregor IA, Wilson ME and Billewicz WZ (1983) Malaria infection of the placenta in The Gambia, West Africa: its incidence and relationship to stillbirth, birthweight and placental weight. *Trans Royal Society of Trop Med and Hygiene.* **77**: 232–44.

93 Gülmezoglu AM and Garner P (1997) Interventions to prevent malaria during pregnancy in endemic malarious areas. In: P Garner, H Gelband, P Olliaro, R Salinas, J Volmink and D Wilkinson (eds) *Infectious Diseases Module of the Cochrane Database of Systematic Reviews.* The Cochrane Collaboration (Issue 4). Update Software, Oxford.

94 Martius JA, Steck T, Ochler MK and Wulf KH (1998) Risk factors associated with preterm birth (< 37 + 0 weeks) and early preterm birth (< 32 + 0 weeks): univariate and multivariate analysis of 106 345 singleton births from the 1994 statewide perinatal survey of Bavaria. *Eur J Obstetr, Gynaecol and Repro Biol.* **80**: 183–9.

95 Divers MJ and Lilford RJ (1993) Infection and preterm labour: a meta-analysis. *Contemp Rev Obstetr and Gynaecol.* **5**: 71–81.

96 Hillier SL, Nugent RP, Eschenbach DA, Krohn MA, Gibbs RS, Martin DH *et al.* for the Vaginal Infections and Prematurity Study Group (1995) Association between bacterial vaginosis and preterm delivery of a low birth weight infant. *New England J Med.* **333**: 1737–42.

97 Brocklehurst P, Hannah M and McDonald H (1998) The management of bacterial vaginosis in pregnancy (Cochrane Review). In: The Cochrane Library (Issue 4). Update Software, Oxford.

98 Royce RA, Jackson TP, Thorp JM, Hillier SL, Rabe LK, Pastore LM and Savitz DA (1999) Race/ethnicity, vaginal flora patterns, and pH during pregnancy. *Sexually Transmitted Diseases.* **26**: 96–102.

99 Goldenberg RL, Klebanoff MA, Nugent R, Krohn MA, Hillier SL and Andrews WW for the Vaginal Infections and Prematurity Study Group (1996) Bacterial colonization of the vagina during pregnancy in four ethnic groups. *Am J Obstetr and Gynecol.* **174**: 1618–21.

100 Yim S-F, Lyon DJ, Chung TKH and Haines CJ (1995) A prospective study of the microbiological environment of the genitourinary tract in Hong Kong Chinese women during pregnancy. *Aus & NZ J Obstetr and Gynaecol.* **35**: 178–81.

101 Romero R, Oyarzun E, Mazor M, Sirtori M, Hobbins JC and Bracken M (1989) Meta-analysis of the relationship between asymptomatic bacteriuria and preterm delivery/low birth weight. *Obstetr and Gynecol.* **73**: 576–82.

102 Schieve LA, Handler A, Hershow R, Pershky V and Davis F (1994) Urinary tract infection during pregnancy: its association with maternal morbidity and perinatal outcome. *Am J Public Health.* **84**: 405–10.

103 Smaill F (1998) Antibiotics vs. no treatment for asymptomatic bacteriuria in pregnancy (Cochrane Review). In: The Cochrane Library (Issue 4). Update Software, Oxford.

104 Villar J, Gülmezolglu AM and De Onis M (1998) Nutritional and antimicrobial interventions to prevent preterm birth: an overview of randomized controlled trials. *Obstetr and Gynecol Survey.* **53**: 575–85.

105 Lechtig A, Martorell R, Delgado H, Yarborough C and Klein RE (1976) Effect of morbidity during pregnancy on birth weight in a rural Guatemalan population. *Ecol Food and Nutrition.* **5**: 225–33.

106 Mata LJ (1978) *The Children of Santa Maria Cauqué: a prospective field study of health and growth.* MIT Press, Cambridge.

107 Garner P, Dubowitz L, Baea M, Lai D, Dubowitz M and Heywood P (1994) Birthweight and gestation of village deliveries in Papua New Guinea. *J Trop Pediatrics.* **40**: 37–40.

108 Kramer MS, McLean FH, Eason EL and Usher RH (1992) Maternal nutrition and spontaneous preterm birth. *Am J Epidemiol.* **136**: 574–83.

109 Meis PJ, Goldenberg RL, Mercer BM, Iams JD, Moawad AH, Miodovnik M, Menard MK, Caritis SN, Thurnau GR, Bottoms SF, Das A, Roberts JM and McNellis D (1998) The preterm prediction study: risk factors for indicated preterm births. *Am J Obstetr and Gynecol.* **178**: 562–7.

110 Churchill D, Perry IJ and Beevers DG (1997) Ambulatory blood pressure in pregnancy and fetal growth. *Lancet.* **349**: 7–10.

111 Peters TJ, Golding J, Butler NR, Fryer JG, Lawrence CJ and Chamberlain GVP (1983) *Plus ça change*: predictors of birthweight in two national studies. *Br J Obstetr and Gynaecol.* **90**: 1040–5.

112 Scott A, Moar V and Ounsted M (1981) The relative contributions of different maternal factors in small for gestational age pregnancies. *Eur J Obstetr, Gynecol and Repro Biol.* **12**: 157–65.

113 Read AW and Stanley FJ (1993) Small for gestational age term birth: the contribution of socio-economic, behavioural and biological factors to recurrence. *Paed and Perinatal Epidemiol.* **7**: 177–94.

114 Orr ST, James SA, Miller CA, Barakat B, Daikoku N, Pupkin M, Engstrom K and Higgins G (1996) Psychosocial stressors and low birthweight in an urban population. *Am J Prev Med.* **12**: 459–66.

115 Mavalanker DV, Gray RH and Trivedi CR (1992) Risk factors for preterm and term low birthweight in Ahmedabad, India. *Int J Epidemiol.* **21**: 263–72.

116 Omu AE, Alothman S, Alqattan F, Alfalah FZ and Sharma P (1996) A comparative study of obstetric outcome of patients with pregnancy induced hypertension – economic considerations. *Acta Obstetr et Gynecol Scand.* **75**: 443–8.

117 Fedrick J and Adelstein P (1978) Factors associated with low birth weight of infants delivered at term. *Br J Obstetr and Gynaecol.* **85**: 1–7.

118 Najmi RS (2000) Distribution of birthweights of hospital born Pakistani infants. *J Pakistan Med Assoc.* **50**: 121–4.

119 Sayers S and Powers J (1997) Risk factors for Aboriginal low birthweight, intrauterine growth retardation and preterm birth in the Darwin Health Region. *Aus and NZ J Public Health.* **21**: 524–30.

120 Chenoweth JN, Esler EJ, Chang A, Keeping JD and Morrison J (1983) Understanding preterm labour: the use of path analysis. *Aus and NZ J Obstetr and Gynaecol.* **23**: 199–203.

121 Martikainen AM, Heinonen KM and Saarikoski SV (1989) The effect of hypertension in pregnancy on fetal and neonatal condition. *Int J Gynaecol and Obstetr.* **30**: 213–20.

122 Ni Chuileannain and Brennecke SP (1999) Recent advances in the prediction of preterm labour. *Current Obstetr and Gynaecol.* **9**: 153–7.

123 Feng Liu D, Dickerman LH and Redline RW (1999) Pathologic findings in pregnancies with unexplained increases in midtrimester maternal serum human chorionic gonadotropin levels. *Am J Clin Pathol.* **111**: 209–15.

124 Yaron Y, Cherry M, Kramer RL, O'Brien JE, Hallak M, Johnson MP and Evans MI (1999) Second trimester maternal serum marker screening: maternal serum α-fetoprotein, β-human chorionic gonadotropin, estriol, and their various combinations as predictors of pregnancy outcome. *Am J Obstetr and Gynecol.* **181**: 968–74.

125 Haddad K, Abirached F, Louis-Sylvestre C, Le Bond J, Paniel B-J and Zorn J-R (1999) Predictive value of early human chorionic gonadotrophin serum profiles for fetal growth retardation. *Human Repro.* **14**: 2872–5.

126 Majzoub JA, McGregor JA, Lockwood CJ, Smith R, Taggart MS and Schulkin J (1999) A central theory of preterm and term labor: putative role of corticotropin-releasing hormone. *Am J Obstetr and Gynecol.* **180**: S232–41.

127 Hobel CJ, Dunkel-Schetter C, Roesch SC, Castro LC and Arora CP. Maternal plasma corticotropin-releasing hormone associated with stress at 20 weeks' gestation in pregnancies ending in preterm delivery. *Am J Obstetr and Gynecol.* **180**: S257–63.

128 Erickson K, Thorsen P, Chrousos G, Grigoriadis DE, Khongsaly O, McGregor J and Schulkin J (2001) Preterm birth: associated neuroendocrine, medical and behavioral risk factors. *J Clin Endocrinol and Metab.* **86**: 2544–52.

129 Lockwood CJ (1999) Stress associated preterm delivery: the role of corticotropin-releasing hormone. *Am J Obstetr and Gynecol.* **180**: S264–6.

130 Kramer MS, Goulet L, Lydon J, Séguin L, McNamara H, Dassa C, Platt RW, Chen MF, Gauthier H, Genest J, Kahn S, Libman M, Rozen R, Masse R, Miner L, Asselin G, Benjamin A, Klein J and Koren G (2001) Socio-economic disparities in preterm birth: causal pathways and analysis. *Paed and Perinatal Epidemiol.* **15** (Suppl 2): 104–23.

131 Blondel B, Kogan MD, Alexander GR, Dattani N, Kramer MS, Macfarlane A and Wen SW (2002) The impact of the increasing number of multiple births on the rates of preterm birth and low birthweight: an international study. *Am J Public Health.* **92**: 1323–30.

CHAPTER 5

Social and environmental determinants of birthweight

This chapter deals with the second major group of birthweight determinants – social and environmental factors. As in the preceding chapter, evidence for the impact of these factors on the whole of the birthweight distribution will be reviewed as well as their effects on preterm birth and the lower extreme of the birthweight distribution.

In Chapter 4, I stressed the intimate relationship of biomedical and socio-environmental influences combining in complex biosocial pathways to determine birthweight. However, prior to exploring how these influences combine and contribute to pathways, the evidence for the separate effects of socio-environmental factors on birthweight is reviewed broadly using the classification employed by Kramer[1] in his methodological review of the determinants of low birthweight. Demographic and psychological factors will be discussed first including socio-economic status (SES), marital status, maternal age and maternal stress and psychological factors. Nutritional factors including gestational weight gain, caloric intake, energy expenditure, iron and other minerals, vitamins and trace elements will then be considered followed by the role of antenatal care and toxic exposures such as smoking.

The objective of the chapter is to identify the main socio-environmental determinants that need to be considered in a model of biopsychosocial pathways to birthweight. As in the preceding chapter, no attempt has been made to carry out a systematic or methodological review of the literature but the chapter draws on a wide range of literature to achieve the objective of identifying determinants that are likely to contribute significantly to the model discussed in Chapter 6. Despite the lack of a specific methodology for including papers and weighting their quality, methodological problems in the interpretation of papers cited will be considered. Much of the literature is concerned with the determinants of low birthweight ($< 2500g$) or preterm birth (< 37 weeks' gestation) with a limited literature on the determinants of birthweight across the whole distribution. Conclusions related to the whole birthweight distribution, therefore, are necessarily extrapolated from those related to low birthweight and preterm birth.

Demographic and psychological factors

Socio-economic status

Socio-economic status is not a single easily classifiable factor such as height or weight but is a constellation of factors representing the social context in which individuals and groups live that structures their life chances in such a way that advantages and disadvantages tend to cluster cross-sectionally and accumulate longitudinally.[2] SES is not a direct causal agent in pregnancy but probably acts as a 'distal' agent exerting its effects through mediating proximal biological and environmental variables.[3] It is an example of what Rose[4] described as 'causes of causes'. The SES constellation includes income, education, marital status (at least in the UK and the USA), a range of income proxies such as car ownership, land ownership and, in the case of the UK, housing tenure and advantage/disadvantage of area of residence as measured by aggregate data. The optimum SES measure (i.e. the one which best reflects the extent of SES effect on a specific outcome) will depend on the population studied and the outcome of interest. These issues are revisited in more detail in Chapter 6 as part of the discussion related to constructing biosocial pathways.

Figures 5.1 and 5.2 show the relationship of birthweight to ecological SES measures in the West Midlands health region of the UK[5] and the Swedish city of Göteborg.[6]

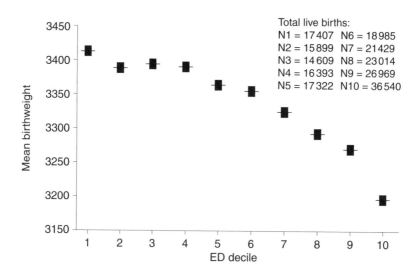

Figure 5.1: Mean birthweight for all live births by enumeration direct (ED) decile ranked by Townsend Deprivation Index, West Midlands Health Region, 1991–93.

Source: Spencer, p. 166.[5]

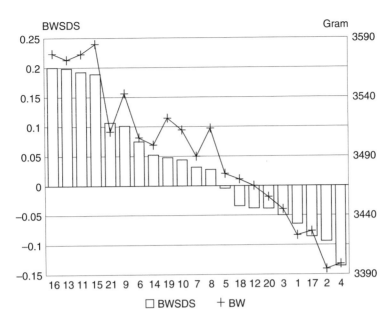

BWSDS

Gram

Figure 5.2: The rank ordered distribution of mean birthweight for gestational age (BWSDS) (score) in the 21 local areas in the city of Göteborg 1982–86, indicated by their respective official numbers, and mean birthweight (BW) (grams) overlaid.

Source: Elmén, p. 150.[6]

The West Midlands health region study,[7] based on 208 567 live births in 1991–93, used a census-based ecological SES measure, the Townsend Deprivation Index (TDI).[8] The TDI, constructed on proportion of unemployed of working age, rented housing, households without access to a car and overcrowding, was calculated for each enumeration district (ED), a collection of about 100 house-holds, and these were aggregated and ranked into deciles by level of deprivation (1 = least deprived and 10 = most deprived). The Göteborg study, reporting on 22 000 singleton births (live and stillbirths) in 1982–86, used a socio-economic area index derived from four indicators (percentage of skilled and unskilled workers; average income men 25–49 years; participation in the last general election; single parents with children under 16 years of age) applied to the 21 administrative areas of the city.

Figures 5.1 and 5.2 show a remarkably similar pattern of finely graded decrease in mean birthweight with increasing disadvantage of the area. Figure 5.2 shows that, in the Swedish sample, this gradient was independent of gestational age as the birthweight standard deviation score (BWSDS) follows the same fine graded pattern. The difference in mean birthweight between most advantaged and most disadvantaged areas was 220g in the West Midlands and 191g (145g for BWSDS) in Göteborg. However, mean birthweights were approximately

200g higher in the Swedish city compared with the West Midlands with the result that the most advantaged area in the West Midlands had a mean birthweight only 30g higher than the most disadvantaged Göteborg area. A study of live singleton births in the northern English city of Sheffield from 1985–94[9] reported the same social patterning of birthweight with a birthweight difference of 170g between the most and least deprived area deciles. This study showed an increase in mean birthweight over the ten-year period of 34g compared with 107g in the 8 years, 1973–81, reported from Göteborg.

Table 5.1: Mean birthweight by SES in developed and less-developed countries

SES in developed countries	Mean birthweight (g)	SES in less-developed countries	Mean birthweight (g)
Britain (1970)[10]		**Morocco (1979)[14]**	
Social class I	3380	Socio-economic level:	
Social class II	3366	High	3392
Social class III nm	3341	Medium	3280
Social class III m	3299	Low	3070
Social class IV	3249		
Social class V	3219		
Unmarried	3143		
Czech Republic (1989–91)[11]		**Thailand (1994–5)[15]**	
University education	3371	Income (Baht):	
Secondary	3350	20 001+	3150
Vocational	3308	10 001–20 000	3121
Primary	3165	5001–10 000	3076
Sweden (1989–91)[11]		⩽ 5000	3064
University education	3570		
Secondary	3526		
Vocational	3545		
Primary	3458		
Netherlands (1981–85)[12]		**Malaysia (1945–76)[16]**	
Income (Gilders):		Income in year prior to birth	
⩾ 36 000	3472	(currency not stated):	
28–36 000	3311	6000+	3210
22–27 999	3376	4000–5999	3140
< 22 000	3221	3000–3999	3120
Norway (1978–82)[13]		2000–2999	3105
Years of education:		1000–1999	3090
> 15	3496	< 1000	3050
13–15	3472		
10–12	3441		
< 10	3371		

Sources: Rush and Cassano, p. 250;[10] Koupilová *et al.*, pp. 11–12;[11] Mackenbach, p. 214;[12] Arntzen, p. 93;[13] Boutaleb, p. 68;[14] Tuntiseranee, p. 627;[15] Da Vanzo *et al.*, p. 394.[16]

The SES gradient in birthweight noted in Figures 5.1 and 5.2 using ecological SES measures is replicated in studies in developed countries[10–13] and less-developed countries based on a range of individual level SES measures (*see* Table 5.1).[14–16]

The consistency of the social gradient across countries suggests powerful influence of social context on birthweight although it does not explain the mechanisms by which the gradient arises. Possible mechanisms are considered in detail in Chapter 6. However, it should be noted that, whatever SES measure was used, a finely graded stepwise decrease in birthweight was found with decreasing SES (*see* Figures 5.1 and 5.2, and Table 5.1).

A few studies have quantified the SES impact on birthweight in regression models including a range of other variables. A Swedish study,[17] using data on 4685 live singleton births at the Akademiska University in Uppsala between 1920–24 and data on 13 918 live singleton births recorded on the Swedish Medical Birth Registry for November and December 1985, showed that infants born to unskilled labourers had an unadjusted reduction in birthweight compared with higher and middle non-manual social class infants of 94g (95% CI 30,158) in 1920–24 and 67g (95% CI 38,97) in 1985. Adjustment for age, parity, gender and gestational age in both cohorts had a marginal effect on the birthweight difference (86g (95% CI 30,142) in 1920–24 and 53g (95% CI 27,80) in 1985). However, adding smoking and height into the 1985 model (measures not available into the 1920–24 model) eliminated the difference. A similar finding was reported in a 10% sample of Quebec births in 1970–71.[18] Each additional year of education was responsible for an increase of 5.76g in birthweight after adjustment for gestational age, maternal pre-pregnancy weight and height, smoking, gender, age and parity.

A Scottish study, using an ecological SES measure, reported a difference in mean birthweight of approximately 170g between the most and least deprived areas but this difference was greatly reduced once smoking, maternal age and height had been taken into account.[19] Comparing regression models fitted on birthweight in the 1958 and 1970 British birth cohorts, Peters *et al.*[20] showed that the determinants of birthweight remained consistent between the cohorts and concluded 'we are unlikely to alter the conclusion that once maternal smoking, height, pre-eclampsia and parity have been taken into account, social class is of relative unimportance in the determination of birthweight' (p. 1044).

These studies[17–20] all demonstrate that adjustment for socially-related variables such as smoking, height, weight, parity and gestational age eliminates the social gradient in birthweight. However, these results do not necessarily support the conclusions of Peters *et al.*[20] They are also consistent with the concept of SES as a distal factor exerting its effect through mediating variables as suggested by Kramer *et al.*[3] and discussed in detail in Chapter 6.

The impact of social factors on low birthweight, intrauterine growth retardation (IUGR) and preterm birth has been extensively studied. Kramer *et al.*[3]

Table 5.2: Continued

Population and year [ref]	SES measure	Preterm birth (%)	IUGR (%)	Low birthweight (%)
Sweden (1989–91)[11]	Maternal education:			
	Primary	6.4		
	Vocational	5.5		
	Secondary	4.9		
	University	4.5		
US Whites (1988)[26]	Income (% poverty level):			
	< 100%	3.5	10.6	6.5
	100–199%	4.7	9.8	4.8
	⩾ 200%	3.4	7.4	3.6
	Maternal education:			
	< 12 years	4.5	11.6	7.5
	12 years	3.9	10.0	4.3
	13–15 years	3.8	5.6	3.9
	⩾ 16 years	2.8	7.5	3.4
US Blacks (1988)[26]	Income (% poverty level):			
	< 100%	12.2	16.7	12.1
	100–199%	9.4	12.9	8.7
	⩾ 200%	7.4	15.9	8.8
	Maternal education:			
	< 12 years	12.0	19.8	13.8
	12 years	12.0	16.7	10.8
	13–15 years	7.5	14.5	9.1
	⩾ 16 years	6.7	9.3	7.0

*Preterm low birthweight.
**Term low birthweight.

Other studies in sub-national populations and population sub-groups show the same gradient.[27–31] A case-control study across 15 European countries[32] involving 1675 preterm births ⩽ 32 weeks' gestation and 3652 births 33–36 weeks' gestation and 7965 unmatched controls showed gradients by education, marital status and social class for birth ⩽ 32 weeks' gestation and 33–36 weeks' gestation. The odds ratios for birth ⩽ 32 weeks' gestation associated with all three social variables were higher than for births at 33–36 weeks' gestation, an observation supported by Kramer et al.[30] in their Montreal study. Both these studies[30,32] reported attenuated but significant social gradients when other factors were adjusted. Other authors[33] have suggested that adjustment for other risk factors eliminates the gradient in preterm birth. The gradient in low birthweight among Danish women, although attenuated, remained significant even when adjusted for age and smoking[22] as did the gradient in term low birthweight among Cardiff women after adjustment for demographic and medical factors and smoking.[28] Results from the limited number of studies from developing countries are consistent with the social patterning of low birthweight, IUGR and preterm birth seen in developed countries. Figure 5.3 shows the distribution of low birthweight (< 2500g) and high birthweight (≥ 3500g) by SES in four rural Guatemalan villages.[34]

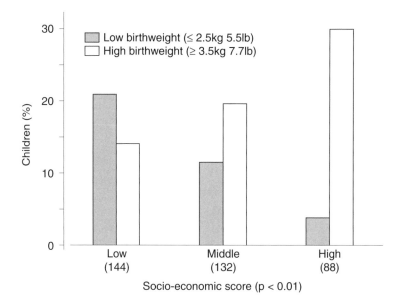

Figure 5.3: Relationship between socio-economic score and proportion of children with low and high birthweights in four rural Guatemalan villages (number of cases given in parentheses; total number is 364).

Source: Lechtig *et al.*, p. 435.[34]

A Brazilian study from São Paulo State reported a prevalence of low birthweight of 7–9.5% among working class families compared with 2.8–3.9% among 'bourgeoisie' classes.[35] SES was also reported to be an important determinant of low birthweight in Karnataka State of South India[36] and of IUGR in Brazil.[37] Both term and preterm low birthweight were associated with low maternal education before adjustment for other factors in a study in Ahmedabad, western India.[38] After adjustment for a range of demographic, obstetric and cultural factors, term, but not preterm, low birthweight remained significant.

The evidence linking birthweight within the 'normal' range with increased risk of adverse childhood (*see* Chapter 1) and adult (*see* Chapter 2) outcomes has led to the concepts of optimal (3500–4500g) and sub-optimal birthweight (< 3500g). The impact of social factors on birthweight can be more fully understood by studying these outcomes. The absolute difference in the proportion of Sheffield infants born < 3500g in the most and the least deprived deciles over the period (1985–94) was 12.5%.[9] If the proportion of births $\geqslant$ 3500g found in the least deprived decile (40%) had been the same for the whole population, then there would have been 9.6% more births within the range associated with better childhood and adult outcomes. Data on births in Scotland in 1978 showed 41.3% of births to social class I mothers in the range $\geqslant$ 3500g compared with 28.3% to social class V mothers.[39] Dowding[40] reporting on 20 698 singleton Greater Dublin births showed a linear relationship of births in the range 3001–4499g with social class. The same patterning was seen in the Guatemalan study[34] illustrated in Figure 5.3.

Confirmation of the role of SES in the determination of birthweight is provided by a Danish study of the effects of decline in SES on the risk of having a low birthweight infant.[41] All women who had a low birthweight infant (< 2500g) and a subsequent liveborn infant in Denmark between 1980 and 1992 and a random sample of the population who gave birth to an infant weighing $\geqslant$ 2500g and to a subsequent liveborn infant were included in the study. The risk of a subsequent low birthweight infant increased after the birth of a first low birthweight infant but deterioration in SES further increased the risk. Among women who had not previously had a low birthweight infant, a decline in SES increased the risk of having a low birthweight infant. Conversely, in both study groups, a rise in SES was associated with a reduced risk of low birthweight in subsequent pregnancies. Using a similar study designed to investigate the impact of changing SES on subsequent preterm birth, the same authors reported that social decline was associated with a moderate increase in the risk of recurrent preterm birth.[42]

Supporting evidence for the role of socio-economic factors in pregnancy outcome comes from two further sources. The Gary Indiana controlled trial of income maintenance that involved an increase in income during pregnancy for women in the intervention group reported a decrease in low birthweight rate among those in the intervention arm and an increase in maternal weight gain in pregnancy.[43] Bhatia and Katz[44] estimated the magnitude of health improvements associated with a proposed living wage ordinance in San Francisco using published observational models of the relationship of income to health. They predicted that a living wage of $11 per hour would be associated with a reduced risk of early childbirth.

Maternal age

Data from studies in developed and less-developed countries suggest that birthweight has a J-shaped relationship with maternal age (see Table 5.3). Both maternal age < 20 and > 34 tend to be associated with a reduction in mean birthweight.

Table 5.3: Mean birthweight by maternal age group in selected countries

Country and year [ref]	Maternal age groups	Mean birthweight (g)	
Scotland 1992–94[19]		**Parity 0**	**Parity ≥ 1**
	≤ 16	3262	3096
	17–19	3259	3276
	20–24	3297	3365
	25–29	3344	3452
	30–34	3333	3484
	35–39	3275	3445
	40–44	3175	3402
	≥ 45	3111	3280
Sweden (Uppsala) 1987[45]			
	15–19	3374	
	20–24	3471	
	25–29	3590	
	30–34	3582	
	35–44	3555	
USA (Alabama) 1983–88[46]		**Non-smoker**	**Smoker**
(all ethnic groups)	≤ 16	3078	3069
	17–19	3161	3088
	20–25	3244	3099
	26–30	3314	3055
	31–35	3305	3024
	≥ 36	3370	3119
Czech Republic 1989–91[11]			
	< 20	3212	
	20–24	3303	
	25–29	3359	
	30–34	3354	
	35–39	3310	
	40+	3250	
Sweden 1989–91[11]			
	< 20	3406	
	20–24	3483	
	25–29	3529	
	30–34	3357	
	35–39	3541	
	40+	3495	
Norway 1978–82[13]			
	< 20	3391	
	20–35	3435	
	>35	3319	
Thailand (Songkhala) 1994–95[15]			
	≤ 20	2995	
	21–25	3116	
	26–30	3090	
	31–35	3139	
	36+	3084	

Sources: Koupilová *et al.*, pp. 11–12;[11] Arntzen *et al.*, p. 57;[13] Tuntiseranee *et al.*, p. 626;[15] Bonellie, p. 20;[19] Nordström and Cnattingius, p. 57;[45] Wen *et al.*, p. 55.[46]

A few studies have attempted to quantify the effect of maternal age on birthweight. A Finnish study[47] reports an increase in birthweight of 36.7g (95% CI 0.7,72.7) for women aged 21–35 years compared with those ⩽ 20 years and an increase of 60.3g (95% CI 12.7,107.9) for women > 35 years after adjustment for other major birthweight determinants. The expected reduction in birthweight with age > 35 is not reported in this study. Three other studies[10,18,48] failed to show any significant effect of maternal age on birthweight after adjustment in a linear regression model although some of the effect of maternal age may have been attenuated in two of the studies[10,18] by the treatment of maternal age as a continuous variable with a linear rather than J-shaped relationship with birthweight.

Kramer[1] concluded in his 1987 methodological literature review 'maternal age does not appear to be an important independent determinant of intrauterine growth retardation or gestational duration. Although age, and particularly very young age, may exert indirect effects by influencing height, weight, nutrition, cigarette smoking as well as alcohol and drug abuse, no direct causal effects can be demonstrated' (p. 682). In Kramer *et al.*'s recent paper on social disparities in pregnancy outcome,[3] the pie diagrams of significant determinants of IUGR and preterm birth do not include maternal age suggesting an unchanged assessment of the impact of maternal age on these outcomes.

Two studies[49,50] published since Kramer's initial review[1] that satisfactorily met (SM) or partially met (PM) his methodological standards (pp. 670–1) for studies of the impact of maternal age (population based and adjusted for ethnicity, height, weight, parity, gestational weight gain, caloric intake, smoking and alcohol) suggest a significant independent role for young maternal age in the determination of low birthweight. A further study[28] fails to show an independent effect of young maternal age on low birthweight but does show an effect of maternal age 35+. Six studies[32,49–53] broadly meeting Kramer's criteria for SM or PM studies report an independent effect of maternal age on preterm birth although a study from Montreal[30] shows no effect after adjustment for a range of confounding variables.

Kramer[1] (p. 681) points out that maternal age may have an indirect impact on pregnancy outcome through its effect on maternal height, weight, gestational nutrition, smoking and alcohol use. Thus it may act in a similar way to SES as a distal cause (*see above* and Chapter 6). Some of the studies published since 1984 suggest that some of the effect of maternal age may be direct and independent of these other factors. However, it is likely that these effects are small with little influence on birthweight and gestational duration.

Stress and maternal psychological factors

Interest in the potential role of stress and psychological factors in the determination of birthweight and gestational duration has increased in recent years motivated by the quest for a better understanding of ethnic and social differences in birth outcomes.[3,54] Further impetus comes from the recognition of possible links between stress, raised levels of placental corticotrophin-releasing hormone and preterm delivery (*see* Chapter 4).[55,56] The terminology related to stress tends to be confusing and incompletely standardised.[54] Here, the classification used by Hoffman and Hatch (p. 381)[54] is broadly followed: 'stressors' describes objective events, acute or chronic, that occur to individuals; 'stress' describes the perception or recognition that an insult has occurred; 'distress' describes negative emotional states that may result from the perception of stress.

Newton and Hunt[57] reported a gradient in mean birthweight by frequency of objective major life events (stressors) in both smoking and non-smoking women in a study of 250 Manchester women in 1980–82 (*see* Table 5.4).

Table 5.4: Mean birthweight among smokers and non-smokers by frequency of major life events

Frequency of objective major life events during pregnancy	Mean birthweight (SD) among non-smokers (g)	Mean birthweight (SD) among smokers (g)	Mean birthweight (SD) among whole sample (g)
No life events	3460 (470)	3140 (540)	3400 (500)
1 life event	3390 (450)	3010 (750)	3260 (600)
⩾ 2 life events	3360 (730)	2890 (890)	3120 (850)

Source: Newton and Hunt, p. 1193.[57]

Among a hospital-based sample of 90 Californian women, each unit increase in a prenatal life events stress score (computed by summing the product of frequency and subjective severity of the life events occurring since the beginning of pregnancy) was associated with a birthweight reduction of 55.03g after adjustment for biomedical risk factors.[58] The score had a possible range of 0–14.7 units. Neither prenatal pregnancy anxiety nor perceived stress were associated with birthweight reduction. A larger study among 842 black and 381 white low income multiparous women in Birmingham, Alabama[59] predicted that a woman with a psychosocial status score (measured between 24 and 32 weeks' gestation) at the 90th percentile would deliver an infant weighing 112–8g less than a woman with a score at the 10th percentile after adjustment for major confounding variables. Other studies[60–63] using a range of measures of stressors, stress and distress report a reduction in birthweight. Aarts and Vingerhoets,[64] however, failed to show any relationship between stressors and birthweight.

Kramer[1] in his 1987 methodological review failed to find any evidence for an association of maternal psychological factors and intrauterine growth. However, a more recent but less methodologically systematic literature review[54] concluded that 'contrary to expectations, psychosocial factors appear to relate more often to fetal growth than to preterm birth' (p. 396). Further, this review identified intimate social support provided by a partner or close family member as an important factor promoting fetal growth independent of the woman's level of stress. This latter finding is contrary to the conclusions of the Cochrane review of random controlled trials (RCTs) of social support in pregnancy[65] but, as Hoffman and Hatch[54] point out, this may be because the interventions in the trials included in the review mainly consisted of professional or stranger rather than intimate support. Although there is little convincing evidence that acute life stressors adversely affect fetal growth,[54] chronic stressors have received less attention[66] and there is some evidence that they may be associated with reduced birthweight.[60,67] Chronic stressors, such as poor housing conditions, debt and unemployment, may be particularly important in explaining social disparities in pregnancy outcomes[3] and are considered further as potentially important components of biopsychosocial pathways in Chapter 6.

Two studies,[68,69] published since the literature reviews,[1,54,66] report a direct effect of psychosocial factors on IUGR independent of potential confounding variables. A prospective cohort study of 872 women giving birth in the city of Malmö, Sweden[68] reported an odds ratio of small for gestational age (> 2 SD below the mean weight for gestational age) of 1.7 (95% CI 0.9,3.3) for women with poor social stability, 2.2 (95% CI 1.1,4.4) for women with poor social participation, 2.6 (95% CI 1.2,5.7) for women with poor instrumental support and 1.5 (95% CI 0.8,2.8) for women with poor emotional support after adjustment for demographic, lifestyle and anthropometric factors. A smaller prospective study of 396 nulliparous Dutch women[69] reported an association of number of hours of housekeeping/week in the first trimester (OR 1.59 (95% CI 1.03,2.46)) and depressed mood in the first trimester (OR 1.12 (95% CI 1.01,1.24)) with small for gestational age ($\leqslant 10^{th}$ Dutch birthweight centile) after controlling for maternal weight and height, smoking and educational level. However, a Scandinavian study[70] of 1552 women reported no relationship between low birthweight and serious life events, stress associated with poor relationship with partner, anxiety or depression.

Hoffman and Hatch[54] report inconclusive evidence for an indirect effect of stressors or distress through lifestyle factors on birthweight. A subsequent study[71] using structural equation modelling reports that stress has no direct influence on birthweight but exerts its effect through addictive behaviour (smoking, alcohol and drug abuse). Figure 5.4 a and b shows the pathways from economic stress to poor social support and family stress through addictive behaviour to low birthweight.

Literature reviews of the impact of maternal psychosocial factors on preterm birth and gestational duration have reached inconsistent conclusions. Kramer's 1987 review[1] concluded that there was a possible effect on preterm

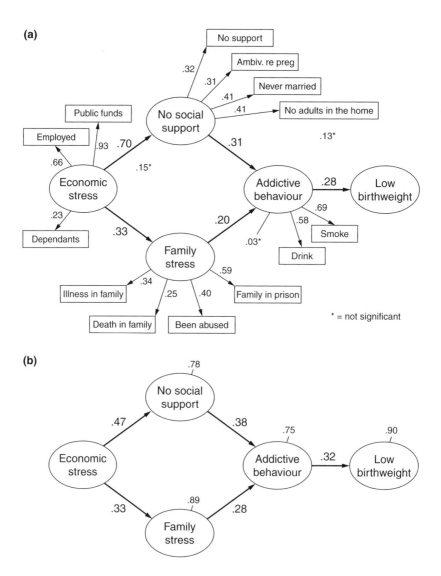

Figure 5.4: (a) Structural equation model of stress factors affecting low birthweight; **(b)** best model of influence of stress factors on low birthweight.

Source: Sheehan, pp. 1508–9.[71]

birth although not on gestational duration. Paarlberg *et al.*'s 1995 review[66] does not specifically address preterm birth or gestational duration as an outcome but does suggest 'it is tempting to hypothesize that stressful situations can potentiate preterm contractions and may trigger preterm labour, especially in the later phases of pregnancy' (p. 580). Hoffman and Hatch[54] found little evidence of a relationship between preterm birth and maternal psychosocial factors but a review in 2000[72] cites major well-designed Scandinavian studies[73,74] suggesting a significant relationship between preterm birth and life events perceived as stressful. A more methodologically robust systematic review[75] of observational studies linking psychosocial factors with preterm birth shows suggestive though not conclusive evidence that stress is related to preterm delivery and mediates between SES and preterm delivery and stronger evidence that job stress, measured by job control and demand, is related to preterm birth. A further study[76] among 739 low income black women published since our systematic review[75] reports an adjusted OR for preterm delivery of 1.86 (95% CI 1.21,2.86) associated with a stress score in the upper quartile on the Prenatal Psychosocial Profile Hassles Scale. A limitation of this study was the collection of stress data after delivery.

In summary, the relationship between maternal psychological factors and preterm birth remains in doubt although there is some indication that particular types of stressor may be implicated. However, as mentioned above, interest in the biochemical mechanisms underlying preterm delivery has prompted renewed interest in the possible role of stress that is currently under investigation in at least two large studies.[56,77]

Demographic and psychological factors and birthweight

- A finely graded stepwise increase in birthweight with increasing socio-economic status has been noted in all countries in which it has been studied.
- Low birthweight, IUGR and preterm birth show a similar gradient.
- Birthweight has a J-shaped relationship with maternal age with lower birthweight at both ends of the age range.
- The evidence for the impact of psychological factors on birthweight and gestational duration is conflicting but some studies do suggest a role of chronic stress in reducing fetal growth and shortening gestational duration.

Nutritional factors in pregnancy and birthweight

This section briefly reviews the extensive evidence base related to the influence of nutritional factors in pregnancy (gestational weight gain, caloric intake, energy consumption, iron deficiency and other specific nutritional deficiencies). The focus of the nutritional debate in relation to birthweight has been the index pregnancy but it is important to recognise that maternal pre-pregnancy weight and height (discussed in Chapter 4) are partly determined by the mother's nutritional status in childhood and prior to conception. The importance of maternal nutrition viewed in this life course perspective to an understanding of pathways to birthweight will be considered further in Chapter 6.

Gestational weight gain

Luke et al.[78] reported mean birthweights for non-smokers and smokers by different levels of gestational weight gain (*see* Table 5.5). Among both non-smokers and smokers there was a stepwise relationship between maternal gestational weight gain and mean birthweight but the effect of smoking on birthweight was noted to be greater among women who gained least weight during pregnancy.

Table 5.5: Mean birthweight among smokers and non-smokers by maternal gestational weight gain

Maternal weight gain (lb)	Non-smoking mean gestational birthweight (95% CI) (g)	Smoking mean birthweight (95% CI) (g)
0–15	3179 (3079,3279)	2936 (2784,3088)
16–25	3173 (3093,3253)	3002 (2848,3156)
26–35	3356 (3286,3426)	3232 (3058,3406)
36+	3491 (3406,3576)	3397 (3209,3585)

Kramer[1] estimated an increase in birthweight of 20.3g per kilogram total gestational weight gain among well-nourished women adding that the effect is likely to be greater among less well-nourished women in developing countries. A study of 2789 adolescent pregnancies (12–19 years of age)[79] fitted regression models on birthweight by weight gain at 12, 16, 20, 24, 28, 32 and 36 weeks' gestation. Controlled for gestation at delivery, ethnicity, maternal pre-pregnancy body mass index, smoking, age and parity, inadequate weight gain (below the lower limit of the 'standard curve' of a published schedule of gestational weight gain at each gestational age) at 12 weeks' gestation was associated with a 10.83g birthweight reduction, at 16 weeks' gestation an 85.77g reduction, at 20 weeks' gestation a 143.40g reduction and 183.38g at 24 weeks' gestation, remaining at this level until term.

Kramer[1] estimated a relative risk of IUGR retardation for a total gestational weight gain of less than 7kg of 1.98. The population attributable risk associated with mean gestational weight gain of 6kg was 36.6% and 13.6% associated with mean gestational weight gain of 11kg (p. 694). Based on meta-analysis of

25 data sets providing information on over 111 000 births worldwide in the WHO Collaborative Study of Maternal Anthropometry and Pregnancy Outcomes, Kelly *et al.*[80] reported an OR of 4.0 (95% CI 3.2,4.8) for IUGR associated with a low attained weight at 28 weeks' gestation among mothers with below average pre-pregnancy weight. For all mothers, the risk for IUGR of low attained weight at 28 weeks' gestation was 3.0 (95% CI 2.7,3.3). Early (conception to 24 weeks' gestation) inadequate weight gain among adolescent pregnancies increased the risk of IUGR by 2.85 (95% CI 1.82,4.47) and late (24 weeks' gestation to term) inadequate weight gain increased the risk by 2.17 (95% CI 1.41,3.34).[81] Inadequate weight gain in both periods of pregnancy was associated with a risk of IUGR of 4.33 (95% CI 2.58,7.26).

The relationship of poor maternal weight gain and preterm birth is less clear. Kramer[1] failed to find any convincing evidence of gestational weight gain influencing gestational duration. However, a later critical review of observational studies[82] concluded that a lower rate of weight gain in pregnancy is associated with an increased risk of preterm delivery and that a slow rate of gain during the latter part of pregnancy may be particularly important. Three subsequently reported studies[83–85] support the association of a low rate of gestational weight gain with preterm delivery although two[83,84] suggest that high rates of weight gain as well as low rates carry an increased risk of preterm delivery. The third study[85] reported an interaction between low pre-pregnancy body mass index (BMI) and a low rate of gestational weight gain during the second and third trimesters resulting in a higher risk of spontaneous preterm birth. These authors also noted an increased risk of spontaneous preterm birth among smokers whose pre-pregnancy weight was low.

Caloric and protein intake and energy consumption

Maternal undernutrition, characterised by inadequate intake of calories, protein and other nutrients, combined with heavy physical work is the single most important cause of low birthweight globally.[86] In countries where undernutrition is highly prevalent, low birthweight forms part of a life course continuum of inadequate nutrition perpetuated through generations (*see* Figure 5.5).

Maternal undernutrition manifests itself through short stature, low pre-pregnancy weight and inadequate gestational weight gain. As considered above, these factors remain powerful determinants of birthweight in developed countries despite the low prevalence of undernutrition. However, there is continuing debate around the value of nutritional interventions during pregnancy in the prevention of adverse pregnancy outcomes in developed countries.

Gestational weight gain is the outward manifestation of the combination of caloric and protein intake and energy consumption. It is easier to measure[1] and has tended for this reason to be the main nutritional measure used in

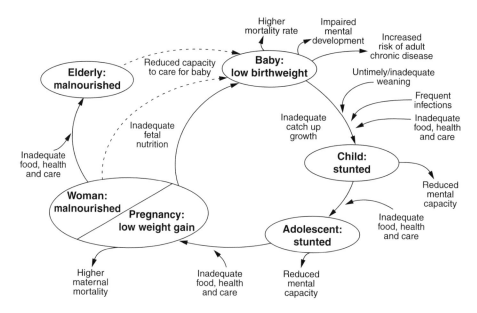

Figure 5.5: Nutrition throughout the life cycle.

Source: Podja and Kelly, p. 2.[86]

observational studies of pregnancy outcomes. Caloric and protein intake, however, are readily tested in controlled clinical trials, the source of much of the best evidence related to their impact on pregnancy outcomes. Evidence related to energy consumption, usually through work, comes from observational studies.

Kramer[1] summarised the results of studies of caloric supplementation and estimated that 100kcal/day supplement throughout pregnancy was associated with a birthweight increase of 99.7g among undernourished women and 34.6g among well-nourished women. Caloric supplementation has no effect on gestational duration but 100kcal/day throughout pregnancy is associated with a reduced risk of IUGR of 0.47 among undernourished and 0.82 among well-nourished women. Kramer[1] concluded that there was 'no evidence for an important role for maternal protein intake or status in either gestational duration or intrauterine growth retardation'. (p. 698)

In later, more methodologically exacting systematic reviews of well designed RCTs of balanced protein/energy supplementation (balanced refers to a supplement in which protein accounts for < 25% of the total energy content) Kramer[87,88] revised his initial assessment concluding that balanced energy/ protein supplementation modestly improves fetal growth (weighted mean difference from 12 RCTs 30g (95% CI 1,58)) but is unlikely to be of long-term benefit to pregnant women or their infants. Despite this definitive conclusion, the controversy related to supplementation continues. An RCT among chronically undernourished women in rural Gambia[89] reported a reduced risk of low birth-weight associated with supplementation with high energy groundnut biscuits for 20 weeks before delivery of 0.58 (95% CI 0.39,0.86) in the hungry season and 0.64 (95% CI 0.45,0.90) in the harvest season. Observational studies in developed countries continue to produce contradictory results. Mathews et al.,[90] based on a study in Portsmouth, UK, concluded that maternal nutrition had little effect on birthweight in industrialised countries. Others[91] challenged this conclusion citing a dose-response relationship between nutrient intake and birthweight in a socially disadvantaged population in Hackney, London.[92]

Kramer[1] was unable to reach a definitive conclusion on the impact of maternal work on either gestational duration or intrauterine growth. Part of the difficulty was the failure in many studies to distinguish between work involving high energy consumption or fatigue associated with standing for long periods and more sedentary work. A further problem is the failure to account for domestic or housework that may lead to fatigue as readily as paid employment. Kramer[1] suggested that future studies should distinguish between the effects of energy expenditure, posture, fatigue and stress.

In their recent paper Kramer et al.[3] allocate a small proportion of their pie diagram depicting the determinants of preterm birth to strenuous work and prolonged standing, stressing that only a small percentage of women are exposed to these conditions. However, they acknowledge that physically demanding domestic work may make a larger contribution. Work is not included in the major determinants of IUGR in Kramer et al.'s paper.[3] A small effect of prolonged standing,[93,94] working late into pregnancy[93] and working long hours[94,95] on small for gestational age births has been noted although others[96,97] have reported that the effects disappear on controlling for socio-economic confounders.

Physical work especially among women in less developed countries may play a larger part in the determination of pregnancy outcomes but present evidence does not allow clear conclusions to be reached.

Iron, anaemia and other specific nutritional deficiencies

Iron deficiency anaemia is the commonest specific nutritional deficiency worldwide. It has a high prevalence in the Indian sub-continent and is closely associated with poverty. In developed countries it is found most commonly in poor women and children and migrants of Indian sub-continental origin. However, exploration of the impact of iron deficiency anaemia is complicated by a number of factors: frequent lack of information about pre-pregnancy iron status;[1] the normal haematological changes (fall in haemoglobin levels, reaching a nadir in the second trimester and rising again to term) occurring in response to plasma volume expansion during pregnancy;[98] haemoglobin levels may not fully reflect maternal iron stores.[99] As a consequence of these difficulties,

Kramer[1] concluded that 'studies that have a bearing on the impact of iron or anaemia on intrauterine growth or gestational duration are particularly weak from a methodological standpoint' (p. 699). Later reviews[98,99] have identified similar problems in observational studies related to the effects of iron on pregnancy outcome.

Few studies have reported the impact of iron on mean birthweight. An Indian study in urban and rural areas of the Punjab[100] reported mean birthweights of 2.23kg among women with a haemoglobin < 7g/dL, 2.65kg among those with a haemoglobin of 7–10.9g/dL compared with 3.25kg among non-anaemic women (Hb ⩾ 11g/dL). Haemoglobin levels were estimated at different times during pregnancy and no attempt was made to adjust for potential confounding variables such as calorie intake. The effects of haemoglobin in the higher range (> 13g/dL) were not investigated perhaps because there were very few women in this population with high levels.

A UK-based study[101] reported quite different results among 115 176 'white' women (*see* Table 5.6). Haemoglobin concentrations ⩽ 85g/dL were associated with a small reduction in mean birthweight but the greatest effect on mean birthweight was seen in those women with haemoglobin concentrations in the upper range. A J-shaped relationship of birthweight was demonstrated with a haemoglobin concentration of 86–95g/dL (well within the normally recognised anaemic range) being associated with the highest level of birthweight. The authors suggest that failure of the haemoglobin concentration to fall below 105g/dL indicates an increased risk of reduced birthweight although this conclusion has been challenged.[102–104]

Table 5.6: Mean birthweight, low birthweight and preterm birth rates by haemoglobin concentration among UK 'white' women

Haemoglobin concentration (g/dL)	Mean birthweight (SD) (g)	Proportion < 2500g (%)	Proportion born at < 37 weeks' gestation (%)
⩽ 85 (n = 499)	3381 (674)	7.8	9.6
86–95 (n = 3185)	3483 (565)	3.8	5.2
96–105 (n = 17 411)	3461 (522)	3.2	3.9
106–115 (n = 40 614)	3413 (518)	3.8	4.5
116–125 (n = 34 671)	3347 (541)	5.3	5.7
126–135 (n = 11 072)	3265 (590)	8.1	9.0
136–145 (n = 1477)	3179 (640)	11.6	12.1
> 145 (n = 121)	2935 (787)	25.6	22.5

Source: Steer *et al.*, p. 490.[101]

Other studies[105,106] have shown a J-shaped relationship of low birthweight with haemoglobin concentration among different populations in developed countries although these studies reported a higher optimal haemoglobin concentration for birthweight. Lu et al.[107] reported that the relationship of maternal haematocrit < 37% with fetal growth retardation became non-significant once other risk factors were accounted for but the increased risk associated with haematocrit > 40% persisted despite controlling for 'race', parity, age, smoking, hypertension and maternal height and weight. By contrast, a Canadian study[108] reported that although initial haemoglobin was not related to infant birthweight, late antenatal haemoglobin showed a significant inverse relationship. However, these results were not adjusted for the same range of confounding variables as Lu et al.'s study.[107]

The contrasting findings between developing and developed countries may be associated with the huge differences in prevalence of iron deficiency anaemia among women. Consistent with the findings of the Punjab study,[100] a study from a malaria endemic area of Papua New Guinea[109] reported that women with early pregnancy anaemia (< 8g/dL) had a higher prevalence of low birthweight (65%) compared with those with haemoglobin concentrations ≥ 8g/dL (27%). A study from Nepal quoted by Ramakrishnan et al.[98] also reported a relationship of low haemoglobin concentration with low birthweight as well as demonstrating the J-shaped relationship with haemoglobin concentrations reported in studies from developed countries.

The evidence linking haemoglobin concentration to preterm delivery suggests a similar J-shaped relationship,[53,101,105–107] although the relationship adjusted for confounding variables was non-significant for lower concentrations in two of the studies.[53,107] An earlier study[110] of 12 718 Boston women giving birth between August 1977 and March 1980 reported very different findings – statistically significant increases in prematurity were noted at all haematocrit levels ≤ 38% and risk of preterm birth was lowest among women with haematocrits between 41–44%. This study failed to show a J-shaped relationship.

Experimental studies of iron supplementation show inconsistent results that are marred by small sample sizes, lack of blinding and poor accounting for other confounding factors.[98] Two RCTs with iron supplementation from Finland[111] and Denmark[112] did not show any significant difference in mean birthweight or rate of low birthweight. An RCT conducted in the Gambia[113] showed a statistically non-significant increase in birthweight of 56g among women supplemented with iron and folate compared with those supplemented with folate alone. A smaller birthweight increase (30g) was noted among Nigerian women receiving iron supplementation compared with those receiving placebo.[114]

Observational studies suggest that low folate status may be associated with impaired fetal growth[115–117] and preterm birth.[117] Experimental studies have produced conflicting results: three RCTs in India,[118] Denmark[119] and France[120] have shown significant increases in birthweight associated with folate supplementation; three other studies in developed countries,[121–123] failed to show any effect on birthweight. Current knowledge would seem to support Kramer's contention[1] that 'evidence supporting an important role for folic acid in intrauterine growth is weak; however, a beneficial effect on folate-deficient populations cannot be entirely ruled out' (p. 700). However, it is intriguing to note that Kramer *et al.*[77] are studying potential genetic pathways from low folate levels in pregnancy to preterm birth in their large case-control study of social disparities in preterm birth.

Recent interest has focused on other micronutrients such as zinc and magnesium. Tamura and Goldenberg[124] identified 22 out of 41 published observational studies that reported a significant association of zinc status with birthweight. Two prospective studies[125,126] among poor urban communities in the USA reported that low serum zinc levels ($< 60\mu g/dL$) in late pregnancy and low zinc intakes ($< 6mg/day$) were associated with increased risk of low birthweight after controlling for energy intakes during pregnancy and other confounding variables. Ramakrishnan *et al.*[98] identified ten experimental trials of zinc supplementation in pregnancy: five trials showed a significant increase in birthweight in the intervention groups. The remaining trials showed no effect. Three trials reported a reduction in preterm delivery associated with supplementation. There appears to be good evidence that zinc status is associated with birthweight and possibly gestational duration and that supplementation may be beneficial.

The evidence for an association of hypomagnesaemia with birthweight and gestational duration remains unclear.[98] Observational studies suggest that magnesium levels were positively associated with an increasing trend in birthweight[127] and a possible association with preterm labour.[128] Experimental studies of magnesium supplementation are inconclusive. A Cochrane systematic review[129] of RCTs of magnesium supplementation found some evidence of an effect on low birthweight and preterm delivery but the positive effects were substantially influenced by two poor quality trials that contributed excessive weight to the analysis. The only 'good quality' trial[130] failed to show any effect of supplementation on pregnancy outcomes. Further higher quality trials investigating pregnancy outcomes were recommended.

A recent report of the possible effect of low consumption of seafood in early pregnancy on preterm delivery and low birthweight[131] raises some interesting possibilities especially in explaining some of the differences in preterm and low birthweight rates among populations in which seafood is expensive and difficult for low income groups to obtain. Among 8729 pregnant women in Aarhus, Denmark, preterm delivery fell progressively from 7.1% in the group never consuming fish to 1.9% in the group consuming fish as a hot meal and open sandwich (a common way of eating fish in Denmark) at least once per week. The risk of low birthweight in the group not eating seafood, adjusted for smoking, alcohol consumption, age, parity, height, pre-pregnant weight, length of education and cohabitant status, was 3.22 (95% CI 1.73,6.00).

The majority of studies of nutrients in pregnancy have examined the influence of single nutrients.[98] However, nutritional deficiencies do not occur in isolation. Although interactions among several micronutrients are known to occur, very little is known about the effect of these interactions on pregnancy outcomes. In addition, very few studies, especially high quality experimental trials, have been undertaken in developing countries among populations most likely to benefit from supplementation. Ramakrishnan et al.[98] recommend further well-designed trials especially in developing countries and examining interactions between micronutrients.

Nutritional factors in pregnancy and birthweight

- An increase in gestational weight of 1kg is associated with an increase in birthweight of 20.3g among well-nourished women in developed countries – the effect among less well-nourished women in developing countries is likely to be greater.
- Evidence for the association of gestational weight gain with gestational duration is conflicting – some recent studies suggest that inadequate and excess gain may both be associated with preterm birth.
- Calorie supplementation increases birthweight but the amount of the increase varies with the level of nourishment of the population – 100kcal/day throughout pregnancy is associated with a birthweight increase of 99.7g among undernourished women and between 30–35g in well-nourished women.
- Calorie supplementation has no effect on gestational duration.
- Physical work especially among women in less-developed countries may play a significant part in the determination of birthweight and gestational duration but present evidence does not allow clear conclusions to be reached.
- Haemoglobin concentration appears to have a J-shaped relationship with birthweight and gestational duration.
- The role of other micronutrients such as zinc and magnesium remains unclear.

Toxic exposures

Smoking

Numerous studies confirm the impact of maternal smoking on infant birthweight. Table 5.7 illustrates the dose-response relationship of smoking with mean birthweight (*see also* Tables 5.4 and 5.5).

Table 5.7: Mean birthweight and smoking in selected countries

Country [ref] and pregnancy smoking category	Mean birthweight (g)						
USA:[132]							
0	3364						
1–10	3189						
11+	3125						
Italy:[133]	**Boys**	**Girls**					
0	3373	3220					
1–9	3266	3132					
$\geqslant 10$	3126	3052					
Sweden:[45]							
Non-smokers	3595						
Occasional smoker	3536						
Regular smoker	3380						
Scotland:[19]	**Parity 0**	**Parity $\geqslant 1$**					
Non-smokers	3387	3354					
Ex-smokers	3380	3516					
Smokers who stop in pregnancy	3292	3427					
Smokers who continue	3149	3228					
England (1986–91):[40]	(Birthweight adjusted to average woman)*						
0	3734						
1–9	3572						
10–19	3510						
$\geqslant 20$	3477						

Britain (1970):[10]	**Registrar General's Social Class**						
	I	**II**	**IIIn–m IIIm**		**IV**	**V**	**Unmarried**
Non-smokers	3403	3416	3360	3362	3311	3313	3245
Stopped before pregnancy	3363	3424	3436	3392	3366	3376	3099
Stopped during pregnancy	3518	3382	3523	3432	3303	3322	3267
< 5 throughout pregnancy	3395	3323	3321	3321	3295	3251	3208
5–14 throughout pregnancy	3282	3252	3237	3187	3153	3128	3034
$\geqslant 15$ throughout pregnancy	3212	3194	3181	3161	3127	3069	3092

*Individualised birthweight ratio multiplied by the mean birthweight of a male infant born at 40 weeks' gestation to a white mother of height 163cm, weight 64kg and parity 1.
Sources: Marbury et al., p. 1167;[132] Conter et al., p. 769;[133] Rush and Cassano, p. 250;[10] Bonellie, p. 22;[19] Dowding, p. 920;[40] Nordström and Cnattingius, p. 57.[45]

These data indicate that smoking is associated with a reduction of mean birthweight of around 200g before controlling for other factors and shows a consistent dose-response relationship. Studies that have estimated the effects of smoking on birthweight adjusted for potential confounding variables report birthweight reductions of 72g among black US women,[134] 158g among white US women,[134] 84g among British 1958 births,[20] 93g among British 1970 births,[20] and 135g for under ten cigarettes/day and 148g for ten or more a day among Finnish women.[47] Kramer,[1] based on studies meeting the quality criteria for exploration of the impact of smoking on birthweight, calculated a risk of birthweight reduction of 149g associated with smoking in pregnancy with a reduction of 11g per cigarette smoked per day.

In populations with a high prevalence of smoking in pregnancy (40%), Kramer[1] estimates that smoking carries a population attributable risk for IUGR of 36.2%. In the pie diagram for IUGR included in their recent paper, Kramer et al.[3] allocate just under a quarter of the pie to smoking based on a population in which 25% of women smoke. This reduction in the population attributable risk (PAR) associated with smoking reflects the fall in prevalence of smoking in pregnancy among women in developed countries since the late 1980s. Kramer[1] estimates a relative risk of 2.42 of IUGR associated with smoking in pregnancy. This level of risk is confirmed by a huge study of more than 1 million Swedish births from 1983–96[135] that reported a risk of birthweight < 2500g of 1.60 (95% CI 1.52,1.70) associated with under ten cigarettes/day and 2.15 (95% CI 2.09,2.21) associated with ten or more cigarettes/day and a risk of birthweight for gestational age $\geq$ –2 SD of 2.08 (95% CI 2.02,2.13) and 2.68 (95% CI 2.60,2.76) associated with the same levels of smoking. Smoking in pregnancy is associated with an increased risk of preterm birth although the risk is less than that for IUGR. Kramer[1] estimated a relative risk of preterm birth of 1.41 associated with smoking and calculated a PAR of 14.1% in a population in which 40% of women smoke in pregnancy. Both the risk (approximately 1.3) and the PAR estimates (approximately 10%) are considerably reduced in Kramer et al.'s recent paper.[3] The Swedish study[135] suggests a higher risk of birth < 32 weeks' gestation associated with under ten cigarettes/day (1.41 (95% CI 1.33, 1.49)) and with ten or more cigarettes/day (1.69 (95% CI 1.58,1.80)) but a similar risk as Kramer et al.'s estimate[3] for birth 32–36 weeks' gestation.

Smoking plays a major role in the determination of birthweight especially in developed countries. However, smoking among women in developed countries is increasingly associated with social and material disadvantage and may act as a major mediator of the relationship between SES and pregnancy outcome.[3] The relationship between smoking, SES and birthweight will be discussed in greater detail in the next chapter particularly their roles in the biosocial pathways to birthweight.

Alcohol and other toxic exposures

Consumption of at least two alcoholic drinks/day has been estimated to be associated with a reduction of 155g in birthweight.[1] The risk of IUGR associated with this level of alcohol consumption was estimated as 1.78 although the low prevalence of daily alcohol consumption at this level in pregnancy resulted in a small PAR (2.3%) associated with alcohol.[1] Use of marijuana or cocaine may also restrict fetal growth but their relatively low prevalence keeps the PAR low.[3] Kramer[1] was unable to find any evidence for a significant effect of caffeine/coffee consumption on birthweight. A subsequent study from Brazil confirmed this lack of effect.[136] None of these exposures has been shown to significantly affect gestational duration.

Combined effects of toxic exposures

A small number of studies have examined the combined effects of toxic exposures on birthweight. Peacock et al.[137] reported that women who were heavy smokers ($\geqslant$ 13 cigarettes/day), heavy drinkers ($\geqslant$ 100g/week) and had high caffeine intake ($\geqslant$ 2801mg/week) had a predicted reduction in mean birthweight of 18% (95% CI 11,24). This combined effect was greater than the effects of the exposures alone. A further report based on the same study[138] suggested that caffeine intake, measured by blood caffeine concentrations, is only associated with reduction in birthweight among smokers. Marbury et al.[132] reported that mean birthweight decreased in a stepwise fashion from non-smokers and non-drinkers to heavy smokers and heavy drinkers. The mean birthweight for heavy smoking non-drinkers was 3119g compared with 2919g for heavy smokers and heavy drinkers.

Toxic exposures

- Smoking throughout pregnancy is associated with a reduction in birthweight of 149g with a birthweight reduction of 11g per cigarette smoked per day.

- In populations with high prevalence of smoking in pregnancy (40%), smoking has an estimated PAR for IUGR of 36.2% and 14% for preterm birth.

- Alcohol consumption is associated with an increased risk of IUGR but the PAR is likely to be small because of the low prevalence of heavy drinking.

- Caffeine consumption has little effect on birthweight.

- Smoking and alcohol consumption are likely to have an additive effect on birthweight.

Antenatal care

In his 1987 methodological review, Kramer[1] was unable to reach any definitive conclusions related to the effectiveness of early antenatal care or its frequency or quality on either intrauterine growth or prematurity. He found some evidence of a favourable effect of high quality antenatal care among high risk groups but the evidence generally was too weak to reach definitive conclusions.

Although antenatal care is not included in their pie diagrams for the determinants of IUGR or preterm birth, Kramer et al.[3] report that more recent observational studies[139–141] show strong associations between late entry into antenatal care or gestational-age adjusted number of antenatal care visits and the occurrence of preterm birth. Specially designed preterm prevention programmes[142,143] have also reported positive results in observational studies. However, there is a discrepancy between these findings and those from randomised trials of antenatal care that have failed to show any real effect, even of 'intensive' programmes.[144,145]

The reason for this discrepancy may be related to the implausibility of the components of antenatal care actually influencing the key determinants of preterm birth. Kramer et al.[3] conclude 'the association between the timing or number of prenatal care visits and the risk of preterm birth may have less to do with what is gained from the visits than with confounding psychological differences between women who initiate prenatal care early and visit their obstetrician, family physician or midwife on a regular basis and women who do not' (p. 200).

Chapter summary

- There is a marked social gradient in birthweight, IUGR and preterm birth.
- Maternal age has a J-shaped relationship with birthweight.
- Chronic stress may be associated with low birthweight and shortened gestational duration.
- Gestational weight gain has an impact on birthweight but calorie supplementation has only been shown to have a marginal effect even in poorly nourished populations.
- Haemoglobin concentration has a J-shaped relationship with birthweight and gestational duration but evidence related to other micronutrients remains unclear.
- Smoking is strongly related to birthweight and gestational duration with a high population attributable risk in populations where smoking in pregnancy is common.
- Alcohol is associated with a reduction in birthweight but not gestational duration.
- Despite evidence from observational studies for a positive effect of high quality antenatal care on birthweight and gestational duration, the results of RCTs fail to show any convincing effect.

References

1 Kramer MS (1987) Determinants of low birth weight: methodological assessment and meta-analysis. *Bull WHO.* **65**: 663–737.

2 Bartley M, Blane D and Montgomery S (1997) Health and the life course: why safety nets matter. *BMJ.* **314**: 1194–6.

3 Kramer MS, Séguin L, Lydon J and Goulet L (2000) Socio-economic disparities in pregnancy outcome: why do the poor fare so poorly? *Paed and Perinatal Epidemiol.* **14**: 194–210.

4 Rose G (1992) *The Strategy of Preventive Medicine.* Oxford University Press, Oxford.

5 Spencer NJ (2000) *Poverty and Child Health* (2e). Radcliffe Medical Press, Oxford: p. 155.

6 Elmén H, Höglund D, Karlberg P, Niklasson A and Nilsson W (1996) Birth weight for gestational age as a health indicator: birth weight and mortality measures at a local area level. *Eur J Public Health.* **6**: 137–41 (p. 140).

7 Spencer NJ, Bambang S, Logan S and Gill L (1999) Socioeconomic status and birth weight: comparison of an area-based measure with the Registrar General's social class. *J Epidemiol and Community Health.* **53**: 495–8.

8 Townsend P, Phillimore P and Beattie A (1988) *Health and Deprivation.* Croom Helm, Beckenham.

9 Spencer NJ, Logan S and Gill L (1999) Trends and social patterning of birthweight in Sheffield, 1985–94. *Arch of Disease in Childhood.* **81**: F138–40.

10 Rush D and Cassano P (1983) Relationship of cigarette smoking and social class to birth weight and perinatal mortality among all births in Britain, 5–11 April 1970. *J Epidemiol and Comm Health.* **37**: 249–55.

11 Koupilová I, Vågerö D, Leon DA, Pikhart H, Príkazsky, Holčík J and Bobák M (1998) Social variation in size at birth and preterm delivery in the Czech Republic and Sweden, 1989–91. *Paed and Perinatal Epidemiol.* **12**: 7–24.

12 Mackenbach JP (1992) Health inequalities in the Netherlands. *Soc Sci and Med.* **34**: 213–26.

13 Arntzen A, Samuelson SO, Magnus P, Bakketeig LS (1994) Birth weight related to social indicators in Norway. *Eur J Public Health.* **4**: 92–7.

14 Boutaleb Y, Lahlou N, Oudghiri A and Mesbahi M (1982) Le poids de naissance dans un pays africain. *J de Gynécol, Obstétr et Biol Repro.* **11**: 68–72.

15 Tuntiseranee P, Olsen J, Chongsuvivatwong V and Limbutara S (1999) Socioeconomic and work related determinants of pregnancy outcome in southern Thailand. *J Epidemiol and Comm Health.* **53**: 624–9.

16 DaVanzo J, Habicht J-P and Butz WP (1984) Assessing socioeconomic correlates of birthweight in peninsular Malaysia: ethnic differences and changes over time. *Soc Sci and Med.* **18**: 387–404.

17 Vågerö D, Koupilová I, Leon DA and Lithell U-B (1999) Social determinants of birthweight, ponderal index and gestational age in Sweden in the 1920s and the 1980s. *Acta Paed Scand.* **88**: 445–53.

18 Fabia J (1973) Régression multiple du poids de naissance utilisant dix variables 'prédictives'. *Can J Public Health.* **64**: 548–51.

19 Bonellie SR (2001) Effect of maternal age, smoking and deprivation on birthweight. *Paed and Perinatal Epidemiol.* **15**: 19–26.

20 Peters TJ, Golding J, Butler NR, Fryer JG, Lawrence CJ and Chamberlain GVP (1983) *Plus ça change*: predictors of birthweight in two national studies. *Br J Obstetr and Gynaecol.* **90**: 1040–5.

21 Wilkins R, Sherman GJ and Best PAF (1991) Birth outcomes and infant mortality by income in urban Canada, 1986. *Health Rep.* **3**: 7–31.

22 Helweg-Larsen K, Olsen O and Madsen M (1999) *Births and Social Factors.* DIKE, Copenhagen: p. 41.

23 Olsén P, Läärä E, Rantakillio P, Järvelin M-R, Sarpola A and Hartikainen A-L (1995) Epidemiology of preterm delivery in two birth cohorts with an interval of 20 years. *Am J Epidemiol.* **142**: 1184–93.

24 Sanjose S, Roman E and Deral V (1991) Low birthweight and preterm delivery, Scotland 1981–84: effect of parents' occupation. *Lancet.* **338**: 428–31.

25 Rodriquez C, Regidor E and Gutierrez-Fisac JL (1995) Low birth weight in Spain associated with sociodemographic factors. *J Epidemiol and Comm Health.* **49**: 38–42.

26 Parker JD, Schoendorf KC and Kiely JL (1994) Associations between measures of socio-economic status and low birth weight, small for gestational age and premature delivery in the United States. *Ann Epidemiol.* **4**: 271–8.

27 Read AW and Stanley FJ (1993) Small for gestational age term birth: the contribution of socio-economic, behavioural and biological factors to recurrence. *Paed and Perinatal Epidemiol.* **7**: 177–94 .

28 Meis PJ, Michielutte R, Peters TJ, Bradley Wells H, Evan Sands R, Coles EC and Johns KA (1997) Factors associated with term low birthweight in Cardiff, Wales. *Paed and Perinatal Epidemiol.* **11**: 287–97.

29 Arbuckle TE and Sherman GJ (1989) Comparison of the risk factors for pre-term delivery and intrauterine growth retardation. *Paed and Perinatal Epidemiol.* **3**: 115–29.

30 Kramer MS, McLean FH, Eason EL and Usher RH (1992) Maternal nutrition and spontaneous preterm birth. *Am J Epidemiol.* **136**: 574–83.

31 Reading R, Openshaw S and Jarvis SN (1990) Measuring child health inequalities using aggregations of enumeration districts. *J Public Health Med.* **12**: 160–7.

32 Ancel P-Y, Saurel-Cubizolles M-J, Di Renzo GC, Papiernik E and Bréart G (1999) Very and moderate preterm births: are the risk factors different? *Br J Obstetr and Gynaecol.* **106**: 1162–70.

33 Wildschut HIJ and Golding J (1997) How important a factor is social class in preterm birth? (Letter) *Lancet.* **350**: 148.

34 Lechtig A, Delgado H, Lasky R, Yarbrough C, Klein RE and Habicht J-P and Béhar M (1975) Maternal nutrition and fetal growth in developing societies. *Am J Disease in Childhood.* **129**: 553–6.

35 da Silva AA, Barbieri MA, Bettiol H, Dal Bó CM, Mucillo G and Gomes UA (1991) Perinatal health: low birth weight and social class. *Revue Saude Publica.* **25**: 87–95.

36 Nair NS, Rao RS, Chandrashekar S, Acharya D and Bhat HV (2000) Socio-demographic and maternal determinants of low birth weight: a multivariate approach. *Ind J Pediatr.* **67**: 9–14.

37 Rondó PHC, Abbott R, Rodrigues LC and Tomkins AM (1997) The influence of maternal nutritional factors on intrauterine growth retardation in Brazil. *Paed and Perinatal Epidemiol.* **11**: 152–66.

38 Mavalnakar DV, Gray RH and Trivedi CR (1992) Risk factors for preterm and term low birthweight in Ahmedabad, India. *Int J Epidemiol.* **21**: 263–72.

39 Chalmers I and Macfarlane A (1981) Problems in the interpretation of perinatal mortality statistics. In: D Hull (ed) *Recent Advances in Paediatrics.* pp. 1–12.

40 Dowding VM (1981) New assessment of the effects of birth order and socioeconomic status on birth weight. *BMJ* (Clinical Research Edition). **282**: 683–6.

41 Basso O, Olsen J, Johansen AMT and Christensen K (1997) Change in social status and risk of low birth weight in Denmark: population based cohort study. *BMJ.* **315**: 1498–1502.

42 Basso O, Olsen J and Christensen K (1999) Study of environmental, social and paternal factors in preterm delivery using sibs and half sibs: a population-based study in Denmark. *J Epidemiol and Comm Health.* **53**: 20–3.

43 Kehrer BH and Wolin CM (1978) Impact of income maintenance on low birthweight: evidence from the Gary Experiment. *J Human Res.* **14**: 432–61.

44 Bhatia R and Katz M (2001) Estimation of health benefits from a local living wage ordinance. *Am J Public Health.* **91**: 1398–402.

45 Nordström M-L and Cnattingius S (1996) Effects on birthweights of maternal education, socio-economic status and work-related characteristics. *Scand J Soc Med.* **24**: 55–61.

46 Wen SW, Goldenberg RL, Cutter GR, Hoffman HJ, Cliver SP, Davis RO and DuBard MB (1990) Smoking, maternal age, fetal growth and gestational age at delivery. *Am J Obstetr and Gynecol.* **162**: 53–8.

47 Järvelin M-R, Elliott P, Kleinschmidt I, Martuzzi M, Grundy C, Hartikainen A-L and Rantakillio P (1997) Ecological and individual predictors of birthweight in a northern Finland birth cohort, 1986. *Paed and Perinatal Epidemiol.* **11**: 298–312.

48 Horon IL, Strobino DM and MacDonald HM (1983) Birth weights among infants born to adolescent and young adult women. *Am J Obstetr and Gynecol.* **146**: 444–9.

49 Ketterlinus RD, Henderson SH and Lamb ME (1990) Maternal age, sociodemographics, prenatal health and behavior: influences on neonatal risk status. *J Adolescent Health Care.* **11**: 423–31.

50 Lee MC, Suhng LA, Lu TH and Chou MC (1998) Association of parental characteristics with adverse outcomes of adolescent pregnancy. *Family Practice.* **15**: 336–42.

51 Gardosi J and Francis A (2000) Early pregnancy predictors of preterm birth: the role of a prolonged menstruation-conception interval. *Br J Obstetr and Gynecol.* **107**: 228–37.

52 Olausson PMO, Cnattingius S and Goldberg RL (1997) Determinants of poor pregnancy outcomes among teenagers in Sweden. *Obstetr and Gynecol.* **89**: 451–7.

53 Meis PJ, Michielutte R, Peters TJ, Bradley Wells H, Evan Sands R, Coles EC and Johns KA (1995) Factors associated with preterm birth in Cardiff, Wales: I. Univariable and multivariable analysis. *Am J Obstetr and Gynecol.* **173**: 590–6.

54 Hoffman S and Hatch MC (1996) Stress, social support and pregnancy outcome: a reassessment based on recent research. *Paed and Perinatal Epidemiol.* **10**: 380–405.

55 Lockwood CJ (1999) Stress associated preterm delivery: the role of corticotropin-releasing hormone. *Am J Obstetr and Gynecol.* **180**: S264–6.

56 Rich-Edwards N, Krieger N, Majzoub J, Zierler S, Lieberman E and Gillman M (2001) Maternal experiences of racism and violence as predictors of preterm birth: rationale and study design. *Paed and Perinatal Epidemiol.* **15**: 124–35.

57 Newton RW and Hunt LP (1984) Psychosocial stress in pregnancy and its relation to low birth weight. *BMJ.* **288**: 1191–4.

58 Wadhwa PD, Sandman CA, Porto M, Dunkel-Schetter C and Garite TJ (1993) The association between prenatal stress and infant birth weight and gestational age at birth: a prospective investigation. *Am J Obstetr and Gynecol.* **169**: 858–65.

59 Goldenberg RL, Hickey CA, Cliver SP, Gotlieb S, Woolley TW and Hoffman HJ (1997) Abbreviated scale for the assessment of psychosocial status in pregnancy: development and evaluation. *Acta Obstetr et Gynecol Scand.* **76**: 19–29.

60 Ramsey CN, Abell TD and Baker LC (1986) The relationship between family functioning, life events, family structure, and the outcome of pregnancy. *J Fam Practice.* **22**: 521–7.

61 Molfese VJ, Bricker MC, Manion L, Yaple K and Beadnell B (1987) Stress in pregnancy: the influence of psychological and social mediators in prenatal experiences. *J Psychosomatic Obstetr and Gynaecol.* **6**: 33–42.

62 Lobel M, Dunkel-Shetter C and Scrimshaw SCM (1992) Prenatal maternal stress and prematurity: a prospective study of socioeconomically disadvantaged women. *Health Psychol.* **11**: 32–40.

63 Cliver SP, Goldenberg RL, Cutter GR, Hoffman HJ, Copper RL, Gotlieb SJ and Davis RO (1992) The relationship among psychosocial profile, maternal size, and smoking in predicting fetal growth retardation. *Obstetr and Gynecol.* **80**: 262–7.

64 Aarts MCG and Vingerhoets AJJM (1993) Psychosocial factors and intra-uterine fetal growth: a prospective study. *J Psychosomatic Obstetr and Gynaecol.* **14**: 249–58.

65 Hodnett ED (2000) Support during pregnancy for women at increased risk (Cochrane Review). In: The Cochrane Library (Issue 1). Update Software, Oxford.

66 Paarlberg KM, Vingerhoets AJJM, Passchier J, Dekker GA and Van Geijn HP (1995) Psycho-social factors and pregnancy outcome: a review with emphasis on methodological issues. *J Psychosomatic Res.* **39**: 563–95.

67 Reeb KA, Graham AV, Zyzanski SJ and Kitson GC (1987) Predicting low birthweight and complicated labor in urban black women: a biopsychosocial perspective. *Soc Sci and Med.* **25**: 1321–7.

68 Dejin-Karlsson E, Hanson BS, Östergren P-O, Lindgren A, Sjöberg N-O and Marsal K (2000) Association of a lack of psychosocial resources and the risk of giving birth to small for gestational age infants: a stress hypothesis. *Br J Obstetr and Gynaecol.* **107**: 89–100.

69 Paarlberg KM, Vingerhoets AJJM, Passchier J, Dekker GA, Heinen AGJJ and Van Geijn HP (1999) Psychosocial predictors of low birthweight: a prospective study. *Br J Obstetr and Gynaecol.* **106**: 834–41.

70 Jacobsen G, Schei B and Hoffman HJ (1997) Psychosocial factors and small for gestational age infants among parous Scandinavian women. *Acta Obstetr et Gynaecol Scand.* **165**: 14–8.

71 Sheehan TJ (1998) Stress and low birth weight: a structural modeling approach using real life stressors. *Soc Sci and Med.* **47**: 1503–12.

72 Austin M-P and Leader L (2000) Maternal stress and obstetric and infant outcomes: epidemi-ological findings and neuroendocrine mechanisms. *Aus and NZ J Obstetr and Gynaecol.* **40**: 331–7.

73 Hedegaard M, Henriksen TB, Secher NJ, Hatch MC and Sabroe S (1996) Do stressful life events affect duration of gestation and risk of preterm delivery? *Epidemiol.* **7**: 339–45.

74 Lou HC, Hansen D, Nordentoft M, Pryds O, Jensen F, Nim J and Hemmingsen R (1994) Prenatal stressors of human life affect fetal brain development. *Dev Med and Child Neurol.* **36**: 826–32.

75 Aveyard P, Forster D, Spencer NJ, Manaseki S, Fry-Smith A, Hyde C, Gardosi J and Cheng KK (2002) Does stress cause premature delivery? A systematic review of observational studies. *J Epidemiol and Comm Health* (in press).

76 Misra DP, O'Campo P and Strobino D (2001) Testing a sociomedical model for preterm delivery. *Paed and Perinatal Epidemiol.* **15**: 110–22.

77 Kramer MS, Goulet L, Lydon J, Séguin L, McNamara H, Dassa C, Platt RW, Chen MF, Gauthier H, Genest J, Kahn S, Libman M, Rozen R, Masse R, Miner L, Asselin G, Benjamin A, Klein J and Koren G (2001) Socio-economic disparities in preterm birth: causal pathways and analysis. *Paed and Perinatal Epidemiol.* **15** (Suppl 2): 104–23.

78 Luke B, Hawkins MM and Petrie RH (1981) Influence of smoking, weight gain and pregravid weight for height on intrauterine growth. *Am J Clin Nutrition.* **34**: 1410–7.

79 Scholl TO, Hediger ML, Khoo C-S, Healey MF and Rawson NL (1991) Maternal weight gain, diet and infant birth weight: correlations during adolescent pregnancy. *J Clin Epidemiol.* **44**: 423–8.

80 Kelly A, Kevany J, de Onis M and Shah PM (1996) A WHO collaborative study of maternal anthropometry and pregnancy outcomes. *Int J Gynaecol and Obstetr.* **53**: 219–33.

81 Hediger ML, Scholl TO, Belsky DH, Ances IG and Wexberg Salmon R (1989) Patterns of weight gain in adolescent pregnancy: effects on birth weight and preterm delivery. *Obstetr and Gynecol.* **74**: 6–12.

82 Carmichael SL and Abrams B (1997) A critical review of the relationship between gestational weight gain and preterm delivery. *Obstetr and Gynecol.* **89**: 865–73.

83 Carmichael SL, Abrams B and Selvin S (1997) The association of pattern of maternal weight gain with length of gestation and risk of spontaneous preterm delivery. *Paed and Perinatal Epidemiol.* **11**: 392–406.

84 Schieve LA, Cogswell ME and Scanlon KS (1999) Maternal weight gain and preterm delivery: differential effects by body mass index. *Epidemiol.* **10**: 141–7.

85 Spinillo A, Capuzzo E, Piazzi G, Ferrari A, Morales V and Di Mario M (1998) Risk for spontaneous preterm delivery by combined body mass index and gestational weight gain patterns. *Acta Obstetr et Gynecol Scand.* **77**: 32–6.

86 Podja J and Kelly L (2000) Low birthweight: a report based on the International Low Birthweight Symposium, Dhaka, Bangladesh, June 1999. Nutrition Policy Paper No 18, United Nations Administrative Committee on Coordination/Sub-Committee on Nutrition, New York.

87 Kramer MS (1993) Effects of energy and protein intakes on pregnancy outcome: an overview of the research evidence from controlled clinical trials. *Am J Clin Nutrition.* **58**: 627–35.

88 Kramer MS (1998) Balanced protein/energy supplementation in pregnancy (Cochrane Review). In: The Cochrane Library (Issue 4). Update Software, Oxford.

89 Ceesay SM, Prentice AM, Cole TJ, Foord F, Weaver LT, Poskitt EME and Whitehead RG (1997) Effects on birth weight and perinatal mortality of maternal dietary supplements in rural Gambia: 5 year randomised controlled trial. *BMJ.* **315**: 786–90.

90 Mathews F, Yudkin P and Neil A (1999) Influence of maternal nutrition on outcome of pregnancy: prospective cohort study. *BMJ.* **319**: 339–43.

91 Doyle W, Crawford M and Costeloe K (2000) Maternal nutrition and birth weight. (Letter) *BMJ.* **320**: 941–2.

92 Doyle W, Crawford M, Wynn AHA and Wynn SW (1990) The association between maternal diet and birth dimensions. *J Nutritional Med.* **1**: 9–17.

93 Fortier I, Marcoux S and Brisson J (1995) Maternal work during pregnancy and the risks of delivering a small for gestational age or preterm infant. *Scand J Work, Env and Health.* **21**: 412–8.

94 Peoples-Sheps MD, Siegel E, Suchindran CM, Origasa H, Ware A and Barakat A (1991) Characteristics of maternal employment during pregnancy: effects on low birthweight. *Am J Public Health.* **81**: 1007–12.

95 Tuntiseranee P, Geater A, Chongsuvivatwong V and Kor-anantakul O (1998) The effect of heavy maternal workload on fetal growth retardation and preterm delivery: a study among southern Thai women. *J Occ and Env Med.* **40**: 1013–21.

96 Klebanoff MA, Shiono PH and Carey JC (1990) The effect of physical activity during pregnancy on preterm delivery and birth weight. *Am J Obstetr and Gynecol.* **163**: 1450–6.

97 Teitelman AM, Welch LS, Hellenbrand KG and Bracken MB (1990) Effect of maternal work activity on preterm birth and low birth weight. *Am J Epidemiol.* **131**: 104–13.

98 Ramakrishnan U, Manjrekar R, Rivera J, Gonzáles-Cossío T and Martorell R (1999) Micronutrients and pregnancy outcome: a review of the literature. *Nutrition Research.* **19**: 103–59.

99 Scholl TO and Hediger ML (1994) Anemia and iron-deficiency anemia: compilation of data on pregnancy outcome. *Am J Clinical Nutrition.* **59** (Suppl 1): 492S–501.

100 Sarin AR (1995) Severe anemia of pregnancy, recent experience. *Int J Gynecol and Obstetr.* **50** (Suppl 2): S45–9.

101 Steer P, Alam MA, Wadsworth J and Welch A (1995) Relation between maternal haemoglobin concentration and birth weight in different ethnic groups. *BMJ.* **310**: 489–91.

102 Vause S, Maresh M and Khaled K (1995) Maternal haemoglobin and birth weight in different ethnic groups – methods do not support conclusions. (Letter) *BMJ.* **310**: 1601.

103 Houghton A (1995) Maternal haemoglobin and birth weight in different ethnic groups – study's conclusions are implausible. (Letter) *BMJ.* **310**: 1601.

104 Howe D (1995) Maternal haemoglobin and birth weight in different ethnic groups – lower haemoglobin may be the result rather than the cause of larger fetuses. (Letter) *BMJ.* **310**: 1601.

105 Garn SM, Ridella SA, Petzold S and Falkner F (1981) Maternal Hb levels and pregnancy outcomes. *Seminars in Perinatol.* **5**: 155–62.

106 Murphy JF, O'Riordan J, Newcombe RG, Coles EC and Pearson JF (1986) Relation of haemoglobin levels in first and second trimester to outcome of pregnancy. *Lancet.* **i**: 992–4.

107 Lu ZM, Goldenberg RL, Cliver S, Cutter G and Blankson M (1991) The relationship between maternal hematocrit and pregnancy outcome. *Obstetr and Gynecol.* **77**: 191–4.

108 Higgins AC, Pencharz PB, Strawbridge JE, Maughan GB and Moxley JE (1982) Maternal hemoglobin changes and their relationship to infant birth weight in mothers receiving a program of nutritional assessment and rehabilitation. *Nutrition Res.* **2**: 641–9.

109 Brabin BJ, Ginny M, Sapau J, Gaslme K and Paino J (1990) Consequences of maternal anaemia on outcome of pregnancy in a malaria endemic area of Papua New Guinea. *Ann Trop and Med Parasitol.* **84**: 11–24.

110 Lieberman E, Ryan KJ, Monson RR and Schoenbaum SC (1988) Association of maternal hematocrit with premature labor. *Am J Obstetr and Gynecol.* **159**: 107–14.

111 Hemminki E and Rimpela U (1991) A randomized comparison of routine versus selective iron supplementation during pregnancy. *Am College of Nutrition.* **10**: 3–10.

112 Milman N, Agger AO and Nielsen OJ (1994) Iron status markers and serum erythropoietin in 120 mothers and newborn infants: effect of iron supplementation in normal pregnancy. *Acta Obstetr et Gynaecol Scand.* **73**: 200–4.

113 Menendez C, Todd J, Alonso PL, Francis N, Lulat S, Ceesay S and Boge BM (1994) The effects of iron supplementation during pregnancy given by traditional birth attendants on the prevalence of anaemia and malaria. *Trans Royal Society of Trop Med and Hygiene.* **88**: 590–3.

114 Preziosi P, Prual A, Galan P, Daouda H, Boureima H and Hercberg S (1997) Effect of iron supplementation on the iron status of pregnant women: consequences for newborns. *Am J Clin Nutrition.* **66**: 1178–82.

115 Goldenberg RL, Tamura T, Cliver SP, Cutter GR, Hoffman HJ and Copper RL (1992) Serum folate and fetal growth retardation: a matter of compliance. *Obstetr and Gynecol.* **79**: 719–22.

116 Frelut ML, Courcy P, Christides J-P, Blot P and Navarro J (1994) Relationship between maternal serum folate and foetal hypotrophy in a population with a good socio-economical level. *Int J Vitamin and Nutritional Res.* **65**: 267–71.

117 Scholl TO, Hediger ML, Scholl JI, Khoo C-S and Fischer RL (1996) Dietary and serum folate: their influence on the outcome of pregnancy. *Am J Clin Nutrition.* **63**: 520–5.

118 Iyengar L and Rajalakshmi K (1975) Effect of folate acid supplementation on birth weights of infants. *Am J Obstetr and Gynecol.* **122**: 332–6.

119 Rolshau J, Date J and Kristoffersen K (1979) Folic acid supplement and intrauterine growth. *Acta Obstetr et Gynaecol Scand.* **58**: 343–6.

120 Blot I, Papiernik E, Kalwasser JP, Werner E and Tchernia G (1981) Influence of routine administration of folic acid and iron during pregnancy. *Gynecol and Obstetr Invest.* **12**: 294–304.

121 Giles PFH, Harcourt AG and Whiteside MG (1971) The effect of prescribing folic acid during pregnancy on birth weight and duration of pregnancy: a double-blind trial. *Med J Aus.* **2**: 17–21.

122 Fletcher J, Gull A, Fellingham FR, Pranherd TAJ, Brant HA and Menzies DN (1971) The value of folic acid supplements in pregnancy. *J Obstetr and Gynaecol Br Commonwealth.* **78**: 781.

123 Trigg KH, Rendell EJ, Johnson A, Fellinggham FR and Prankerd TA (1976) Folate supplements during pregnancy. *JRCGP.* **26**: 228–30.

124 Tamura T and Goldenberg RL (1996) Zinc nutriture and pregnancy outcome. *Nutrition Res.* **16**: 139–81.

125 Scholl TO, Hediger ML, Scholl JL, Fischer RL and Khoo C-S (1993) Low zinc intake during pregnancy: its association with preterm and very preterm delivery. *Am J Epidemiol.* **137**: 115–24.

126 Neggers YH, Cutter GR, Alvarez JO, Goldenberg RL, Acton R, Go RCP and Roseman JM (1991) The relationship between maternal serum zinc levels during pregnancy and birthweight. *Early Human Dev.* **25**: 75–85.

127 Ghebremeskal K, Burns L, Burden TJ, Harbige L, Costeloe K, Powell JJ and Crawford M (1994) Vitamin A and related essential nutrient in cord blood: relationships with anthropometric measurements at birth. *Early Human Dev.* **39**: 177–88.

128 Kurzel RB (1993) Is low serum magnesium associated with premature labor? *Ann NY Acad Sci.* **678**: 350–2.

129 Markides M and Crowther CA (1998) Magnesium supplementation during pregnancy (Cochrane Review). In: The Cochrane Library (Issue 4). Update Software, Oxford.

130 Sibai BM, Villar MA and Bary E (1989) Magnesium supplementation during pregnancy: a double-blind randomized controlled clinical trial. *Am J Obstetr and Gynecol.* **161**: 115–9.

131 Olsen SF and Secher NJ (2002) Low consumption of seafood in early pregnancy as a risk factor for preterm delivery: prospective cohort study. *BMJ.* **324**: 447–50.

132 Marbury MC, Linn S, Monson R, Schoenbaum S, Stubblefield PG and Ryan KJ (1983) The association of alcohol consumption with outcome of pregnancy. *Am J Public Health.* **73**: 1165–8.

133 Conter V, Cortinovis I, Rogari P and Riva L (1995) Weight growth in infants born to mothers who smoked during pregnancy. *BMJ.* **310**: 768–71.

134 Goldenberg RL, Cliver SP, Mulvihill FX, Hickey CA, Hoffman HJ, Klerman LV and Johnson MJ (1996) *Am J Obstetr and Gynecol.* **175**: 1317–24.

135 Källén K (2001) The impact of maternal smoking during pregnancy on delivery outcome. *Eur J Public Health.* **11**: 329–33.

136 Santos IS, Victora CG, Huttly S and Carvalhal JB (1998) Caffeine intake and low birth weight: a population-based case-control study. *Am J Epidemiol.* **147**: 620–7.

137 Peacock JL, Bland JM and Anderson HR (1991) Effects on birthweight of alcohol and caffeine consumption in smoking women. *J Epidemiol and Comm Health.* **45**: 159–63.

138 Cook DG, Peacock JL, Feyerabend C, Carey IM, Jarvis MJ, Anderson HR and Bland JM (1996) Relation of caffeine intake and blood caffeine concentration during pregnancy to fetal growth: prospective population based study. *BMJ.* **313**: 1358–62.

139 Kotelchuck M (1994) The adequacy of prenatal care utilization index: its US distribution and association with low birthweight. *Am J Public Health.* **84**: 1486–9.

140 Mustard CA and Roos NP (1994) The relationship of prenatal care and pregnancy complications to birthweight in Winnipeg, Canada. *Am J Public Health.* **84**: 1450–7.

141 Barros H, Tavares M and Rodrigues T (1996) Role of prenatal care in preterm birth and low birthweight in Portugal. *J Public Health Med.* **18**: 321–8.

142 Meis PJ, Ernest JM, Moore ML *et al.* (1987) Regional program for prevention of premature birth in northwestern North Carolina. *Am J Obstetr and Gynecol.* **157**: 550–6.

143 Yawn BP and Yawn RA (1989) Preterm birth prevention in a rural practice. *JAMA.* **262**: 230–3.

144 Mueller-Heubach E, Reddick D, Barnett B and Bente R (1989) Preterm birth prevention: evaluation of a prospective controlled randomized trial. *Am J Obstetr and Gynecol.* **160**: 1172–8.

145 Heins HC, Nance NW, McCarthy BJ and Efird CM (1990) A randomized trial of nurse-midwifery prenatal care to reduce low birth weight. *Obstetr and Gynecol.* **75**: 341–5.

CHAPTER 6

Making sense of the evidence: modelling biopsychosocial pathways to birthweight

The final chapter in Part 2 draws together the evidence from the previous two chapters with the aim of constructing a theoretically justifiable and biologically plausible model of the complex biopsychosocial pathway to birthweight. The next, and final, part of the book explores how the model might contribute to more effective programmes promoting optimum birthweight (*see* Chapter 7) and the research and policy implications of the model (*see* Chapter 8).

Consistent with the germ theory of disease causation[1] much of the epidemiological work related to birthweight aims to identify and isolate the effect of single exposures. Although this approach is useful in identifying exposures with greatest impact on birthweight, it tends to underestimate interaction between exposures, fails to account for indirect as well as direct effects and does not allow pathways from distal to proximal exposures through mediating variables to be explored. In constructing the model in this chapter, attention is given not only to the risk attributable to different exposures but also to the effects of cross-sectional clustering and accumulation over time of multiple risk exposures,[2] intergenerational effects[3] and indirect effects of more distal exposures mediated through proximal variables.[4] No model can hope to fully reflect the complexity of the process by which birthweight is determined within individuals and across populations; however, this approach facilitates movement away from static cross-sectional concepts of birthweight determination towards a more dynamic understanding that might assist in promoting optimal birthweight (*see* Chapter 7).

The first task in drawing together the mass of evidence considered in the two preceding chapters is to identify the variables that need to be considered in modelling biopsychosocial pathways. The evidence for relationships among these variables is then discussed to explore how they may be correlated cross-sectionally and over time and to establish the biological and temporal plausibility of the model components. Before considering examples of models of life course pathways from childhood to adult health and setting out the theoretical framework for the model, the concept of proximal and distal causal factors[5] is discussed drawing on examples from the general literature but focusing specifically on proximal and distal causal factors in the determination of birthweight. The essential components of a theoretical framework for a model of birthweight determination will then be outlined prior to bringing the evidence together and constructing the model.

Variables with a major impact on birthweight

From the evidence reviewed in Chapters 4 and 5, the factors, either acting through intrauterine growth or gestational duration, that should be considered in constructing the model are shown in Table 6.1.

Most of these factors have been consistently shown to affect birthweight and/or gestational duration and many demonstrate a dose-response relationship (*see* Chapters 4 and 5). Kramer *et al.*,[4] based on population attributable risk for each factor, constructed pie diagrams for the determinants of IUGR and preterm birth in developed countries in which 25% of women smoke during pregnancy and a substantial minority are non-white (*see* Figures 6.1 and 6.2).

These diagrammatic representations of the risk attributable to each factor are invaluable in identifying the exposures contributing most to the outcome and guiding public health interventions aimed at modifying adverse pregnancy outcomes. However, as intimated above and discussed in more detail below, they fail to account for accumulation of risk over time or the impact of distal factors exerting their effects through these proximal factors. This approach also tends to encourage the view that interventions directed at individual risk exposures can be effective without addressing the complex interplay of proximal and distal factors. The limitations of such approaches in the promotion of optimal birthweight are discussed in detail in Chapter 7.

In the same way as these variables cannot be treated as independent factors acting at a single point in time, they cannot be treated as having exactly the same properties. Specifically low SES does not itself 'cause' adverse pregnancy outcomes but exerts its influence through mediating variables such as smoking, maternal height and other variables listed in Table 6.1 that have a direct effect on the biological processes leading to adverse outcomes.[4] For these reasons, there are methodological objections to the treatment of SES in epidemiological studies of pregnancy outcome as a variable with equivalent properties to height or weight to be entered into a competing regression model to control for confounding. A conceptual model that, as Kramer *et al.*[4] state 'explicitly acknowledges the existence of causal pathways with aetiological factors operating "upstream" or "downstream" relative to one another rather than simultaneously acting, independent determinants' (p. 196) is required to adequately account for the different properties and temporal relationships of variables contributing to birthweight determination.

Table 6.1: Variables with a major impact on birthweight either directly or through gestational duration

Variable	Likely impact on birthweight/gestational duration
Maternal height	1cm increase in maternal height associated with 7.8g increase in birthweight: effect on gestational duration unclear
Pre-pregnancy weight	1kg increase in maternal weight associated with 9.5g increase in birthweight: approximately 25% increase in preterm birth associated with maternal weight < 54kg
Body mass index (BMI)	Based on a single Finnish study, each unit increase in BMI > 19 associated with 33g increase in birthweight
Maternal birthweight	100g increase in maternal birthweight associated with approximate increase of 20g in infant birthweight
'Race'/ethnicity	Varies with ethnic group but black Americans and those from Indian sub-continent have consistently lower birthweight than those of European origin; black Americans have higher levels of preterm birth
Parity	Parity 0 = −158g; 1 = −19.9g; 2 = +29.5g; 3 = +49.5g; 4+ = +99.2g (some studies suggest a decrease in birthweight beyond parity 5)
Malaria (less-developed countries only)	Decrease in birthweight of approximately 140g
Genital infection	Accounts for 15–20% of preterm birth in developed countries: effect on intrauterine growth retardation (IUGR) unclear
Pregnancy-induced hypertension (PIH) < 20 weeks'	Decrease in birthweight of approximately 116g
PIH without proteinuria in later pregnancy	Decrease in birthweight of approximately 66g
PIH with proteinuria	Decrease in birthweight of approximately 160g
Socio-economic status (SES) (including social class, income, education, maternal age, marital status)	Decrease in birthweight of 120–200g: approximately 30% increase in preterm birth
Gestational weight gain/work	20.3g increase in birthweight for every 1kg increase in weight in pregnancy: role of work in relation to preterm delivery unclear
Micronutrient deficiencies including anaemia	May be important in less-developed countries with high prevalence of anaemia and multiple micronutrient deficiencies: J-shaped relationship of haematocrit and ferritin with birthweight and gestational duration noted in developed countries
Smoking	Approximately 150–200g decrease in birthweight and 30% increase in preterm birth
Stress and psychological factors	Association with birthweight and gestational duration is unresolved but could have indirect effect on birthweight

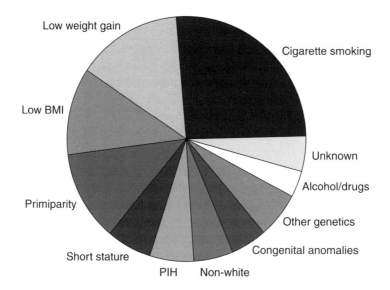

Figure 6.1: Aetiological determinants of IUGR in a developed country in which 25% of the women smoke during pregnancy and a substantial minority are non-white.

Source: Kramer *et al.*, p. 198.[4]

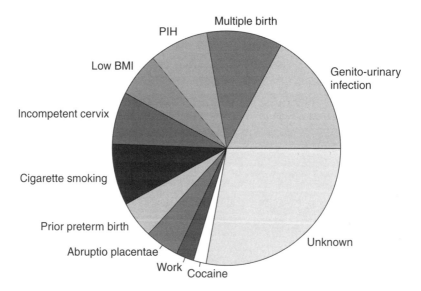

Figure 6.2: Aetiological determinants of preterm birth in a developed country in which 25% of the women smoke during pregnancy and a substantial minority are non-white.

Source: Kramer *et al.*, p. 199.[4]

Relationship between variables impacting on birthweight

Relationships across the life course

Most of the variables listed in Table 6.1 have their origins long before the onset of pregnancy and their inter-relationships are best examined within a life course perspective. Maternal SES of origin has a powerful influence on attained adult height with an adjusted risk of short stature of 2.14 for women of social class IV and V origin compared with those from social classes I and II.[6] In less developed countries, the cycle of malnutrition (*see* Figure 5.5) determines that girls born into poor families will be undernourished in early childhood and come to pregnancy stunted and with a low pre-pregnancy weight.[7,8] Low SES of origin in developed countries is associated with an increased risk of poor early weight gain[9,10] but an increased risk of obesity in adult life.[11]

Maternal birthweight is self-evidently a factor that must be viewed within a life course perspective. It is influenced by the same complex combination of biological, social and environmental factors as infant birthweight and cannot be treated as a purely genetic factor with no social or environmental component.[3,12,13] Maternal birthweight is one means by which biological and social risks are transmitted across generations. There is also evidence that birthweight itself is predictive of future SES so there is likely to be a link between maternal birthweight and her adult SES.[14]

As already discussed in Chapter 4 the use of 'race'/ethnicity in epidemiology is controversial principally because 'race' has been discredited as a genetic entity[15] and ethnicity is constantly changing[16] and is open to misclassification.[17] However, whether the differences in birthweight noted in different ethnic groups are biological or social in origin, it seems clear that ethnicity represents one of the ways in which risk is transmitted across generations. In a life course perspective, black Americans have an elevated risk of experiencing prolonged poverty during childhood and into adulthood,[18] aboriginal Australians are at much higher risk than those of European origin of low income, malnutrition, and growth stunting in childhood and adverse health behaviours in adolescence,[19] and children born to families of Indian sub-continental (ISC) origin (particularly those from Pakistan and Bangladesh) in the UK are more likely to experience prolonged low income in childhood.[20] In addition, these groups are subject to the psychological and material pressures associated with racism.[21] Racism has been suggested as one of the exposures responsible for some of the difference in pregnancy outcomes between black and white Americans possibly exerting its effect through high levels of stress inducing high corticotrophin-releasing hormone levels in pregnancy.[22]

Ethnicity is also associated with other risk factors for poor pregnancy outcome. Aboriginal Australian women come to pregnancy shorter and younger, are more likely to smoke in pregnancy, and have genital tract and urinary tract infections.[23] Black American women are more likely to have genital infections[24,25] and differences in vaginal pH and flora,[25] pregnancy induced hypertension,[26,27] anaemia,[26] and haemorrhage during pregnancy.[27] However, smoking in pregnancy is less common among black American women[26,28] and among women of ISC origin in the UK.[29]

Evidence specifically linking maternal and early childhood factors to PIH is not available. However, as discussed in Chapters 2 and 3, birthweight is associated with increased risk of hypertension in late childhood[30] and early adulthood.[31] It seems reasonable to assume that increased risk of essential hypertension would translate into an increased risk of PIH especially as the birthweight–blood pressure association at 10–11 years is stronger in girls than boys.[30] SES in adulthood is strongly linked to SES of origin whether measured as occupational class,[32] education,[33] or income.[34] Teenage pregnancy,[33] younger age at first pregnancy,[33] and single parenthood[18] are strongly patterned by SES of origin. SES of origin has also been shown to influence micronutrient intake at 36 years of age in the 1946 British national cohort[35] and in middle-aged Finnish men[36] suggesting that the socio-economic life course may be implicated in the nutritional status of women coming to pregnancy in developed as well as developing countries.

Social class differences in smoking among women become established in adolescence and remain entrenched into adulthood.[6] Similar patterns of childhood socio-economic factors influencing smoking behaviour in middle age have been noted in Finnish men.[36] Psychological problems in adulthood have been shown in a number of studies to be associated with childhood SES.[6,36,37] Lundberg[38] has suggested that the effects of childhood SES on adult sense of coherence (an important component of psychological make-up and well-being) are minimal compared with the effects of dissension in the family. Experience of parental divorce and separation in childhood and early adolescence has been shown to increase the risk of psychiatric symptoms in women aged 43 years.[39] Behavioural problems in childhood that are socially patterned[40,41] are known to track into adulthood leading to poor psychological adjustment[42] and contributing to poor job prospects[43] and increased risk of unemployment.[44] Risks acting over the life course are likely to have a cumulative effect over time. For example, it is likely that a female infant born into a poor family in the developing world will be low birthweight, will be more likely to suffer acute illness and poor nutrition leading to stunting, wasting, anaemia and other micronutrient deficiencies and will come to pregnancy early. A similar cumulative trajectory but with modified risk exposures can be postulated for low income women in developed countries: the girl is more likely to have been born low birthweight, to have experienced more childhood ill health, to have had a less nutritious diet with adverse effect on her growth, to have started smoking in adolescence and be less likely to quit in early pregnancy and to come to pregnancy at an earlier age.

Cross-sectional clustering of risk exposures in pregnancy

Clustering of risk exposures in pregnancy has been reported in a number of studies. Kramer *et al.*[4] list the following associations of low SES at the time of pregnancy (p. 202, Table 2): short stature, low gestational weight gain, low intakes of micronutrients, higher rates and quantities of smoking, higher caffeine and alcohol consumption, greater likelihood of prolonged standing and strenuous work, bacterial vaginosis more common, and increased experience of stressful life events, chronic stress and depression. A factor that will work to increase birthweight is BMI that is more likely to be high in low SES women in developed countries.

An association of smoking with gestational weight gain has been reported in a number of studies[45] although it has been suggested that lower fetal weight accounts for most of the difference.[46] Stress, low social support and depression have also been linked to poor gestational weight gain.[45]

Young maternal age, itself linked to SES,[47] has been reported to be associated with low pre-pregnancy weight[48,49] and short stature.[48,50] Smoking and alcohol consumption seem to act synergistically to reduce birthweight.[51,52] The addition of caffeine consumption to smoking and alcohol has been reported to further depress birthweight.[53]

Proximal and distal influences on birthweight

The concept of distal factors exerting their influence through proximal exposures is essential to the construction of biopsychosocial pathways to birthweight. However, this approach to understanding how outcomes are determined over time through mediating variables has been overshadowed by the mass of epidemiological research that treats risk exposures as if they have no temporal relationship to each other and seeks to adjust or control for the effects among covariates. As Lynch *et al.*[36] state

'SES, health behaviours, and psychosocial characteristics are assessed at the same point in time, making it impossible to disentangle the temporal sequencing of SES and these factors. For instance, if social class position in childhood and educational experiences were important in the adoption and maintenance of adult health behaviours, or influential in the development of psychosocial orientations, then it would be inappropriate to "adjust" for these variables, because the SES exposure would be temporally prior to the behaviours and so the behavioural and psychosocial characteristics would be in the causal pathway.' (p. 810)

Although the concept of 'chains of risk' from distal influences in early childhood on late childhood and adult psychopathological outcomes was developed and has been extensively studied by Rutter,[54] life course epidemiology has provided a particular impetus to the approach.[55] The impact of fetal and childhood exposures on adult health mediated through proximal variables such as smoking and nutrition has been studied in relation to adult blood pressure and hypertension,[56] diabetes and insulin action,[57] the acquisition of health capital in adulthood,[58] and premature death.[59]

In discussing socio-economic gradients in health status, Hertzman[60] identifies the period of premature chronic degenerative disease (age period 45–75 years) as the largest component of the gradient and states 'But this is not the time at which the principal determinants of differential mortality and morbidity begin to have their biological effect. It is necessary to work backwards in time to find their origin' (p. 26).[60] As for chronic degenerative disease, so for birthweight. Pregnancy is not an isolated biological process insulated from the rest of the life course – it is a key stage in the life course that brings together the social and biological life course influences and 'chains of risk' carried by the woman and crystallises them into the biological processes that produce the newborn infant.

Maternal height, a key determinant of birthweight, has its origins in the mother's own fetal growth (*see* Chapter 3) and in her early childhood nutritional status (*see above*). Maternal weight is also influenced by early childhood nutrition though less so than height, but maternal obesity appears to be linked to childhood socio-economic status.[11] Micronutrient deficiency, notably iron deficiency, also predates pregnancy in many cases particularly among women in less-developed countries[61] and has its origins in similar early childhood nutritional deficits to maternal height. As discussed above, pregnancy induced hypertension may have part of its origins in the mother's fetal growth. Psychological problems such as depression and chronic stress (*see above*) are established before pregnancy and, like smoking, are influenced by SES in childhood and adolescence.[62] SES in adult life is strongly determined by SES of origin again mediated by early childhood influences on cognitive development[63] and subsequent educational achievement.[33]

Examples of diagrammatic models of pathways to adult health outcomes and to birthweight or gestational duration

Models of life course pathways from infancy/early childhood to adult health

Prior to considering examples of models of pathways to birthweight and/or gestational duration, it is instructive to examine how pathways from infancy/

early childhood to adult health have been represented in the life course literature. One of the most comprehensive models, developed by Power *et al.*[6] to explain inter- and intragenerational relationships between health and circumstances, is shown in Figure 6.3.

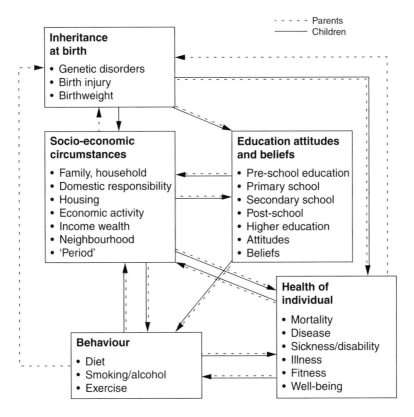

Figure 6.3: Inter- and intragenerational relationships between health and circumstances.

Source: Power *et al.*, p. 23.[6]

This complex model demonstrates the inter-relationship of social, behavioural, genetic and illness factors on health outcomes of parents and their children. The model conveys the intimate relationship between variables influencing health at any point in time and across generations. Of particular interest in the context of this book is the box labelled '"inheritance" at birth'. The authors point out that 'inheritance' includes genetic inheritance, socio-economic circumstances at or prior to birth, and parental health behaviour such as smoking during pregnancy.

In a simpler, less comprehensive model, Kuh *et al.*[64] depict chains of risk from poor childhood socio-economic environment to poor adult health (*see* Figure 6.4).

Their model shows the life course links between poor childhood SES and poor adult health through a range of channels including negative parental or peer role models and inhibition of self esteem and skill development through poor childhood health behaviours and school performance leading to poor adult health behaviours and environment. It is notable that their model links poor SES of origin to teenage pregnancy through skill inhibition leading to poor school performance.

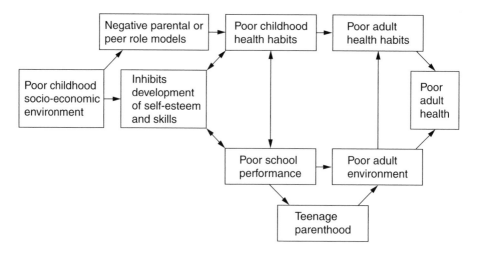

Figure 6.4: Examples of chains of risk.

Source: Kuh *et al.*, p. 177.[64]

Benzeval *et al.*[59] model the relationship between income and health in a life course perspective (*see* Figure 6.5). Their model shows a linear trajectory from childhood circumstances to adult health through transition to adulthood (mainly education) and adult circumstances. Their model encompasses direct and indirect effects but fails to demonstrate the intergenerational continuity of 'inherited' factors shown in Figure 6.4.

Life course influences on respiratory disease are shown in Figure 6.6. This model, based on a presentation by Ben-Shlomo and Kuh[65] and published in Davey Smith *et al.*,[66] is interesting as it demonstrates the accumulation over the life course of social and biological factors impacting on respiratory health in childhood and into adulthood. The bold arrows joining asthmatic tendency or genetic predisposition with infant respiratory infections and these, through childhood chest infections, with adult lung disease represent stronger relationships but these are influenced by the accumulation of negative social risk exposures over the life course.

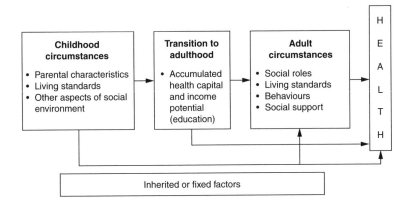

Figure 6.5: Income and health: a life course perspective.

Source: Benzeval *et al.*, p. 98.[59]

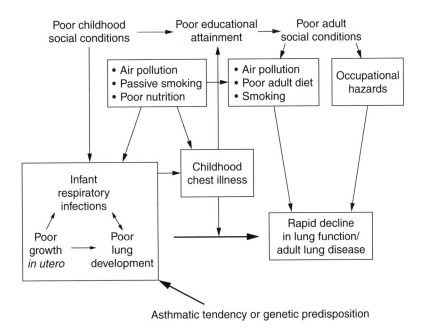

Figure 6.6: Schematic representation of life course influences on respiratory disease.

Source: Davey Smith *et al.*, p. 112.[66]

These models linking 'inherited' and early childhood influences to adult health demonstrate a number of important features of modelling across time that are useful in constructing models of birthweight determination. The different ways of approaching the modelling of life course influences on adult health illustrate the problem of different theoretical constructs underpinning the models. An essential prerequisite in the construction of models is a clear theoretical justification for the proposed model firmly based in empirical work and, where possible, tested in more than one empirical data set. However, the models illustrated above have common features that show the potential power of models in examining pathways and chains of risk over time. These models enable direct and indirect effects to be explored. Cumulative effects of risk exposures acting at different times in the life course can be examined as can the clustering of risks at critical times in the life course. Further, and particularly important in modelling birthweight, they allow the combined effects of social and biological influences to be studied as they exert their influence across generations.

Models of pathways to birthweight and/or gestational duration

Pathway models are unusual in the birthweight and gestational duration literature. Some examples are considered here but none has been found that includes intergenerational influences on birthweight and/or gestational duration. The models are largely confined to the index pregnancy and, in some cases, only include a limited range of predictor variables. One of the most comprehensive is the pathway model of preterm delivery (*see* Figure 6.7) developed using path analysis methods by Chenoweth *et al.*[67]

The factors having a direct independent effect on preterm delivery are represented by bold arrows in the path diagram. Other factors are shown to influence preterm delivery indirectly. Proximal and distal relationships within the index pregnancy are illustrated. The model includes factors that have their origin in the woman's fetal or childhood experience but these relationships are not explored.

Sheehan[68] used a structural equation modelling approach to study the relationship between life stressors and low birthweight. Sheehan's model is shown in Chapter 5, Figure 5.4 a and b (p. 100). Sheehan's path analysis illustrates the importance of exploring potential indirect effects on birthweight. Rutter and Quine,[69] in constructing a diagrammatic model of the relationship between material deprivation and adverse pregnancy outcomes, also postulate direct and indirect effects of stress through adverse health behaviours on pregnancy outcomes (*see* Figure 6.8). Their model includes a pathway through education and cognitive knowledge not included in Sheehan's analysis.

Two other papers present diagrammatic pathways to pregnancy outcome through stress but both of these include the combined effects of psychosocial and biomedical risk factors. Smilkstein *et al.*[70] present a model that does not

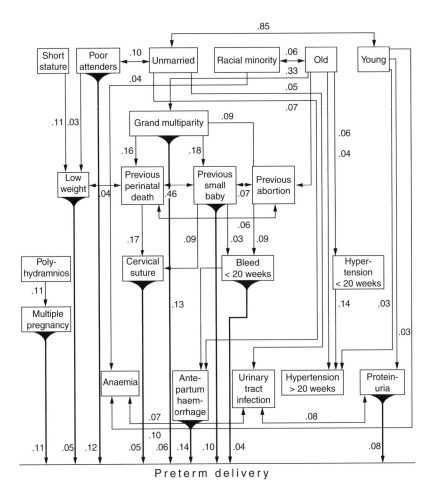

Figure 6.7: Path diagram showing significant positive path coefficients with preterm delivery.

Source: Chenoweth *et al.*, p. 201.[67]

explore direct or indirect effects but simply predicts an additive risk of psychosocial and biomedical factors on pregnancy outcome (*see* Figure 6.9).

Kramer *et al.*[71] construct a more comprehensive and convincing model as part of the design of a study of social disparities in preterm birth (*see* Figure 6.10). Although the model is confined to the index pregnancy, the authors explicitly acknowledge the intergenerational influences on preterm birth and the model combines biological, social and psychological factors to postulate a biopsychosocial pathway to preterm birth. A further intriguing element of this model is the possible link with genetic mutation through low serum folate in social disadvantaged women.

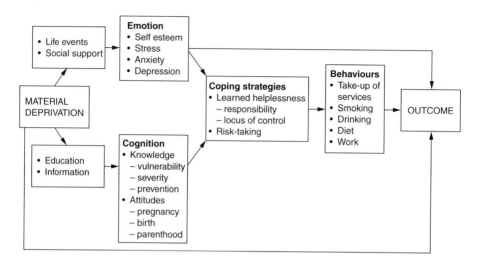

Figure 6.8: A model of psychosocial mediators.

Source: Rutter and Quine, p. 564.[69]

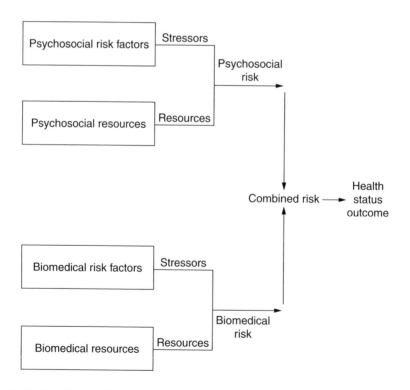

Figure 6.9: Model of biopsychosocial risk factors that influence health status.

Source: Smilkstein *et al.*, p. 316.[70]

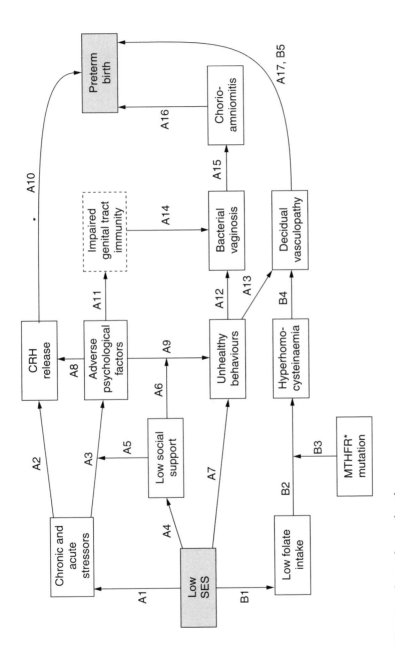

Figure 6.10: Hypothesised causal pathways.

*Methylenetetrahydrofolate reductase.

Source: Kramer *et al.*, p. 110.[71]

These pathway models share one major limitation. Although they include variables with their origins in the mother's own fetal, childhood and adolescent life, all are limited to the index pregnancy. As will be discussed in Chapter 7, this limitation, which these models share with much of the literature on birthweight determination, impedes the development of new approaches to the promotion of optimal birthweight and the prevention of preterm delivery.

Theoretical framework for a model of birthweight determination

I have argued above that an essential prerequisite of pathway models is a clear and explicit theoretical justification and framework. The following is the framework within which the model of birthweight determination presented below (*see* Figure 6.11, p. 140) was constructed.

Biological plausibility

The impact of factors in the model on birthweight either through intrauterine growth or gestational duration must be biologically plausible. The relationships between factors postulated by the model must also be biologically plausible.

Plausible temporal relationships

The temporal relationships postulated in the model must be plausible. Implausible or doubtful temporal relationships should be excluded.

Incorporate major determinants of intrauterine growth and gestational duration

The model must include all the major factors that have been shown to influence intrauterine growth and gestational duration. It is particularly important that the separate contributions of intrauterine growth and gestational duration and their distinct causal pathways to birthweight are incorporated in the model.

Relationships based on sound empirical research

All relationships between predictor variables and birthweight and between predictor variables themselves should be based on sound empirical research.

Empirically testable

The model must be amenable to empirical testing in appropriate data sets. Consistent with path analysis methodology,[72] the model should be tested in more than one data set and, where necessary, alternative model constructions meeting the plausibility criteria should be studied. The objective is to find a biologically and temporally plausible model with the best fit to the data. It should be noted that the relationships depicted in the model presented below (*see* Figure 6.11, p. 140) are based on empirical research but the model itself has yet to be tested in a data set.

Direct and indirect effects

The model should be capable of accounting for direct and indirect effects of predictor variables on birthweight.

Chains of risk

The model must depict the relationship between distal and proximal variables that form chains of risk impacting on birthweight.

Social into biological

Social factors do not have a direct biological effect and cannot 'cause' disturbances of intrauterine growth or gestational duration. Their influence is exerted by the conversion of the social into the biological within individuals. This process should be represented in the model.

Individual and societal level influences on birthweight

The evidence considered so far in this book has largely related to studies carried out on individuals within countries and has been concerned with risks for birthweight and gestational duration within populations. Differences between countries reflecting differences in population, social structures, wealth and political priorities have not been considered and, as Kramer *et al.*,[4] point out variations between countries may not share the same causal explanations. The model presented in this chapter is based on individual level risks in developed countries with ethnically diverse populations. Adaptation of the model to less developed countries would be feasible provided determinants such as malarial infection are included. The role of societal level factors is considered in detail in Chapters 7 and 8 and an adaptation of the model presented that attempts to demonstrate how societal factors might impact on individual risk factors (*see* Figure 7.3, p. 162).

A model of biopsychosocial pathways to birthweight

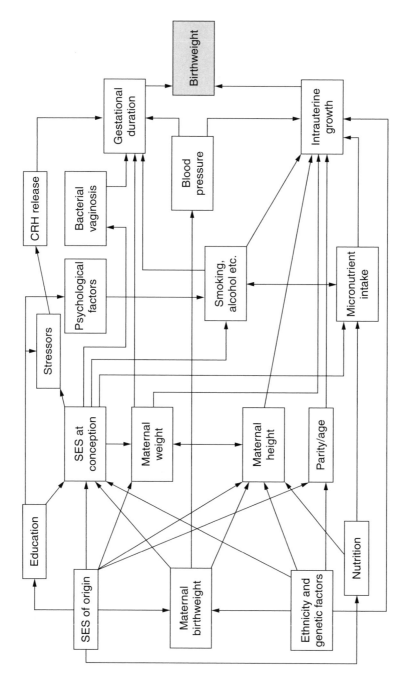

Figure 6.11: Biopsychosocial model of birthweight determination.

Chapter summary

- Risk factors for impaired fetal growth and reduced gestational duration tend to cluster cross-sectionally and accumulate longitudinally.

- Recognition of the temporal sequencing of risk exposures and the relationship of risk exposures to one another over the life course and across generations is essential to understanding the mechanisms by which birthweight is determined – variables need to be analysed as proximal and distal.

- A range of models have been suggested to explain health outcomes taking account of distal and proximal effects but those concerned with birthweight are limited by the scope of the risk exposures considered or by the focus of the outcome on tail of the birthweight or gestational age distribution.

- A theoretical framework for a biopsychosocial model of birthweight determination should fulfil the following: biological plausibility, temporal plausibility, incorporate the major determinants of intrauterine growth and gestational duration, be based on sound empirically proven relationships, be empirically testable, incorporate direct and indirect effects, incorporate chains of risk, and plausibly explain the transformation of the social into the biological.

References

1 Evans AS (1993) *Causation and Disease: a chronological journey*. Plenum Medical Book Company, New York and London.

2 Bartley M, Blane D and Montgomery S (1997) Health and the life course: why safety nets matter. *BMJ.* **314**: 1194–6.

3 Emanuel I, Leisenring W, Williams MA, Kimpo C, Estee S, O'Brien W and Hale CB (1999) The Washington State Intergenerational Study of Birth Outcomes: methodology and some comparisons of maternal birthweight and infant birthweight and gestation in four ethnic groups. *Paed and Perinatal Epidemiol.* **13**: 352–71.

4 Kramer MS, Séguin L, Lydon J and Goulet L (2000) Socio-economic disparities in pregnancy outcome: why do the poor fare so poorly? *Paed and Perinatal Epidemiol.* **14**: 194–210.

5 Rose G (1992) *The Strategy of Preventive Medicine*. Oxford University Press, Oxford.

6 Power C, Manor O and Fox J (1991) *Health and Class: the early years*. Chapman and Hall, London.

7 Podja J and Kelly L (2000) Low birthweight – a report based on the International Low Birthweight Symposium, Dhaka, Bangladesh, June 1999. Nutrition Policy Paper No 18, United Nations Administrative Committee on Coordination/Sub-Committee on Nutrition, New York.

8 WHO Collaborative Study (1995) Maternal anthropometry and pregnancy outcomes. *Bull WHO.* **73** (Suppl 1): 1–98.

9 Wright CM, Waterston A and Aynsley-Green A (1994) Effect of deprivation on weight gain in infancy. *Acta Paed Scand.* **83**: 357–9.

10 Frank DA and Zeisel SH (1988) Failure to thrive. *Pediatric Clinics of North America.* **35**: 1187–205.

11 Parsons T, Power C, Logan S and Summerbell C (1999) Childhood predictors of adult obesity: a systematic review. *Int J Obesity.* **23** (Suppl 8): 1–107.

12 Johnston LB, Clark AJL and Savage MO (2002) Genetic factors contributing to birth weight. *Arch Disease in Childhood.* **86**: Fetal and Neonatal Edition F2–3.

13 Hennessy E and Alberman E (1998) Intergenerational influences affecting birth outcome: I. Birthweight for gestational age in the children of the 1958 British birth cohort. *Paed and Perinatal Epidemiol.* **12** (Suppl 1): 45–60.

14 Power C, Bartley M, Davey Smith G and Blane D (1996) Transmission of social and biological risk across the life course. In: D Blane, E Brunner and R Wilkinson (eds) *Health and Social Organization: towards a health policy for the 21st century.* Routledge, London and New York: pp. 188–203.

15 Lewontin R (1982) *Human Diversity.* Scientific American Books, New York.

16 Nanton P (1992) Official statistics and problems of inappropriate ethnic categorisation. *Policy and Politics.* **20**: 277–85.

17 Spencer NJ (1996) Race and ethnicity as determinants of child health: a personal view. *Child: Care, Health and Dev.* **22**: 327–46.

18 Danziger S and Stern J (1990) *The Causes and Consequences of Child Poverty in the United States.* Innocenti Occasional Papers, No.10. Unicef International Child Development Centre, Florence.

19 Jolly DL (1990) *The Impact of Adversity on Child Health: poverty and disadvantage.* Australian College of Paediatrics, Parkville.

20 Smaje C (1995) *Health, 'Race' and Ethnicity: making sense of the evidence.* King's Fund Institute, London.

21 Kreiger N (2000) Discrimination and health: a US perspective on concepts and measures of epidemiologic studies of health consequences of racism, sexism and other forms of oppression. In: L Berkman and I Kawachi (eds) *Social Epidemiology.* Oxford University Press, Oxford: pp. 36–75.

22 Rich-Edwards J, Krieger N, Majzoub J, Zierler S, Lieberman E and Gillman M (2001) Maternal experiences of racism and violence as predictors of preterm birth: rationale and study design. *Paed and Perinatal Epidemiol.* **15** (Suppl 2): 124–35.

23 Blair E (1996) Why do Aboriginal newborns weigh less? Determinants of birthweight for gestational age. *J Paed and Child Health.* **32**: 498–503.

24 Goldenburg RL, Klebanoff MA, Nugent R, Krohn MA, Hillier S and Andrews WW (1996) Bacterial colonization of the vagina during pregnancy in four ethnic groups. *Am J Obstetr and Gynecol.* **174**: 1618–21.

25 Royce RA, Jackson TP, Thorp JM, Hillier SL, Rabe LK, Pastore LM and Savitz DA (1999) Race/ ethnicity, vaginal flora patterns, and pH during pregnancy. *Sexually Transmitted Diseases.* **26**: 96–102.

26 Goldenberg RL, Cliver SP, Mulvihill FX, Hickey CA, Hoffman HJ, Klerman LV and Johnson MJ (1996) Medical, psychological and behavioural risk factors do not explain the increased risk for low birth weight among black women. *Am J Obstetr and Gynecol.* **175**: 1317–24.

27 Kempe A, Wise PH, Barkan SE, Sappenfield WM, Sachs B, Gortmaker SL, Sobol AM, First LR, Pursley D, Rinehart H, Kotelchuck M, Sessions Cole F, Gunter N and Stockbauer JW (1992) Clinical determinants of the racial disparity in very low birth weight. *NEJM.* **327**: 969–73.

28 Starfield B, Shapiro S, Weiss J, Liang K-Y, Ra K, Paige D and Wang X (1991) Race, family income and low birth weight. *Am J Epidemiol.* **134**: 1167–74.

29 Rudat, K (1994) *Black and Minority Ethnic Groups in England: health and lifestyles.* London: Health Education Authority.

30 Taylor SJC, Whincup PH, Cook DG, Papacosta O and Walker M (1997) Size at birth and blood pressure: cross-sectional study in 8–11 year old children. *BMJ.* **314**: 475–80.

31 Gennser G, Rymark P and Isberg PE (1988) Low birth weight and the risk of high blood pressure in adulthood. *BMJ.* **296**: 1498–500.

32 Johnson P and Reed H (1993) *Two Nations? The Inheritance of Poverty and Affluence.* Institute for Fiscal Studies Commentary No 53. Institute for Fiscal Studies, London.

33 Wadsworth MEJ (1991) *The Imprint of Time.* Clarendon Press, Oxford: pp. 98–113.

34 Kuh D and Wadsworth MEJ (1991) Childhood influences on adult male earnings in a longitudinal study. *Br J Sociol.* **42**: 537–55.

35 Braddon FEM, Wadsworth MEJ, Davies JMC and Cripps HA (1988) Social and regional differences in food and alcohol consumption and their measurement in a national birth cohort. *J Epidemiol and Comm Health.* **42**: 341–9.

36 Lynch JW, Kaplan GA and Salonen JT (1997) Why do poor people behave poorly? Variation in adult health behaviours and psychosocial characteristics by stages of the socioeconomic lifecourse. *Soc Sci and Med.* **44**: 809–19.

37 Wadsworth MEJ and Kuh DJL (1997) Childhood influences on adult health: a review of recent work from the British 1946 national birth cohort study, the MRC National Survey of Health and Development. *Paed and Perinatal Epidemiol.* **11**: 2–20.

38 Lundberg O (1997) Childhood conditions, sense of coherence, social class and adult ill health: exploring their theoretical and empirical relations. *Soc Sci and Med.* **44**: 821–31.

39 Rodgers B (1990) Adult affective disorder and early environment. *Br J Psychiatry.* **157**: 539–50.

40 Ross DP and Roberts P (1999) *Income and Child Well-being: a new perspective on the poverty debate.* Canadian Council on Social Development, Ottawa.

41 Department of Health (1998) *The Health of Young People 1995–97.* The Stationery Office, London.

42 Scott S. Aggressive behaviour in childhood (1998) *BMJ.* **316**: 202–6.

43 Fergusson DM and Horwood LJ (1998) Early conduct problems and later life opportunities. *J Child Psychol and Psychiatry.* **39**: 1097–108.

44 Montgomery SM, Bartley MJ, Cook DG and Wadsworth MEJ (1996) Health and social precursors of unemployment in young men in Great Britain. *J Epidemiol and Comm Health.* **50**: 415–22.

45 Hickey CA (2000) Sociocultural and behavioral influences on weight gain during pregnancy. *Am J Clin Nutrition.* **71** (Suppl 1): S1364–70.

46 Rantakallio P and Hartikainen-Sorri A-L (1981) The relationship between birth weight, smoking during pregnancy and maternal weight gain. *Am J Epidemiol.* **113**: 590–5.

47 Spencer NJ (1993) Teenage mothers. *Current Paediatrics.* **4**: 48–51.

48 Scholl TO, Decker E, Karp RJ, Greene G and De Sales M (1984) Early adolescent pregnancy: a comparative study of pregnancy outcome in young adolescents and mature women. *J Adolescent Health Care.* **5**: 167–71.

49 Zuckerman B, Alpert JJ, Dooling E, Hingson R, Kayne H, Morelock S and Oppenheimer E (1983) Neonatal outcome: is adolescent pregnancy a risk factor? *Pediatrics.* **71**: 489–93.

50 Horon IL, Strobino DM and MacDonald HM (1983) Birth weights among infants born to adolescent and young adult women. *Am J Obstetr and Gynecol.* **146**: 444–9.

51 Marbury MC, Linn S, Monson R, Schoenbaum S, Stubblefield PG and Ryan KJ (1983) The association of alcohol consumption with outcome of pregnancy. *Am J Public Health.* **73**: 1165–8.

52 Wright JT, Waterson EJ, Barrison IG *et al.* (1983) Alcohol consumption, pregnancy and low birthweight. *Lancet.* **8326(i)**: 663–5.

53 Peacock JL, Bland JM and Anderson HR (1991) Effects on birthweight of alcohol and caffeine consumption in smoking women. *J Epidemiol and Comm Health.* **45**: 159–63.

54 Rutter M (1988) Longitudinal data in the study of causal processes: some uses and pitfalls. In: M Rutter (ed) *Studies of Psychosocial Risk: the power of longitudinal data.* European Science Foundation, Cambridge University Press, Cambridge: pp. 29–44.

55 Kuh D and Ben-Shlomo Y (1997) Introduction. In: D Kuh and Y Ben-Shlomo (eds) *A Life Course Approach to Chronic Disease Epidemiology.* Oxford University Press, Oxford.

56 Whincup P and Cook D (1997) Blood pressure and hypertension. In: D Kuh and Y Ben-Shlomo (eds) *A Life Course Approach to Chronic Disease Epidemiology.* Oxford University Press, Oxford: pp. 121–41.

57 McKeigue P (1997) Diabetes and insulin action. In: D Kuh and Y Ben-Shlomo (eds) *A Life Course Approach to Chronic Disease Epidemiology.* Oxford University Press, Oxford: pp. 78–100.

58 Blane D (1999) The life course, the social gradient and health. In: M Marmot and RG Wilkinson (eds) *Social Determinants of Health.* Oxford University Press, Oxford.

59 Benzeval M, Dilnot A, Judge K and Taylor J (2000) Income and health over the lifecourse: evidence and policy implications. In: H Graham (ed) *Understanding Health Inequalities.* Open University Press, Buckingham and Philadelphia.

60 Hertzman C (1999) Population health and human development. In: DP Keating and C Hertzman (eds) *Developmental Health and the Wealth of Nations.* The Guilford Press, New York and London: pp. 19–40.

61 Ramakrishnan U, Manjrekar R, Rivera J, Gonzáles-Cossío T and Martorell R (1999) Micronutrients and pregnancy outcome: a review of the literature. *Nutrition Res.* **19**: 103–59.

62 Brown GW (1988) Causal paths, chains and strands. In: M Rutter (ed) *Studies of Psychosocial Risk: the power of longitudinal data.* European Science Foundation, Cambridge University Press, Cambridge: pp. 285–314.

63 Brooks-Gunn J, Duncan GJ and Britto PR (1999) Are socioeconomic gradients for children similar to those for adults? Achievement and health of children in the United States. In: DP

Keating and C Hertzman (eds) *Developmental Health and the Wealth of Nations*. The Guilford Press, New York and London: pp. 94–124.

64 Kuh D, Power C, Blane D and Bartley M (1997) Social pathways between childhood and adult health. In: D Kuh and Y Ben-Shlomo (eds) *A Life Course Approach to Chronic Disease Epidemiology*. Oxford University Press, Oxford: pp. 169–98.

65 Ben-Shlomo Y and Kuh D (1999) Life course approach to chronic disease. Presentation at: Synthetic Biographies: State of the art and developments. International Workshop, Pisa.

66 Davey Smith G, Gunnell D and Ben-Shlomo Y (2001) Life-course approaches to socio-economic differentials in cause-specific adult mortality. In: D Leon and G Walt (eds) *Poverty, Inequality and Health: an international perspective*. Oxford University Press, Oxford: pp. 88–124.

67 Chenoweth JN, Esler EJ, Chang A, Keeping JD and Morrison J (1983) Understanding preterm labour: the use of path analysis. *Aus and NZ J Obstetr and Gynaecol*. **23**: 199–203.

68 Sheehan TJ (1998) Stress and low birth weight: a structural modeling approach using real life stressors. *Soc Sci and Med*. **47**: 1503–12.

69 Rutter DR and Quine L (1990) Inequalities in pregnancy outcome: a review of psychosocial and behavioural mediators. *Soc Sci and Med*. **30**: 553–68.

70 Smilkstein G, Helsper-Lucas A, Ashworth C, Montano D and Pagel M (1984) Prediction of pregnancy complications: an application of the biopsychosocial model. *Soc Sci and Med*. **18**: 315–21.

71 Kramer MS, Goulet L, Lydon J, Séguin L, McNamara H, Dassa C, Platt RW, Chen MF, Gauthier H, Genest J, Kahn S, Libman M, Rozen R, Masse R, Miner L, Asselin G, Benjamin A, Klein J and Koren G (2001) Socio-economic disparities in preterm birth: causal pathways and analysis. *Paed and Perinatal Epidemiol*. **15** (Suppl 2): 104–23.

72 Vasconcelos AGG, Almeida RMV and Nobre FF (1998) The path analysis approach for multivariate analysis of infant mortality data. *Ann Epidemiol*. **8**: 262–71.

Implications for promotion of optimal birthweight, research and policy

CHAPTER 7

Approaches to promoting optimal birthweight

Part 3 builds on the previous two parts, particularly Chapter 6, to explore approaches to promoting optimal birthweight. Consistent with the evidence presented in Part 1, the focus is on the optimal birthweight range rather than the more common focus on preventing low birthweight ($<$ 2500g) or preterm delivery ($<$ 37 weeks' gestation). Promoting birthweight within the optimal range entails similar challenges of preventing infants being born too early and too small but goes beyond the lower extremes to address ways of shifting the birthweight distribution to the right taking more infants into the optimal range.

This chapter starts by revisiting the concept of an optimal birthweight range considered in Chapters 1 and 2, followed by a detailed examination of the reasons for the relative lack of success of strategies to prevent low birthweight and preterm birth. Alternative approaches at the individual and population level based on the biopsychosocial model of pathways to birthweight (*see* Figure 6.11, p. 140) are explored. An expanded version of the biopsychosocial model incorporating societal level influences on individual characteristics is presented as part of the exploration of alternative preventive strategies. The translation of these promotional approaches into health and social policy is considered in the final chapter of the book.

The concept of an optimal birthweight range

The concept of an optimal range for birthweight arises from the J-shaped pattern of increased risk of a range of infant, childhood and adult outcomes associated with birthweight such that risk is increased up to 3500g, is lowest between 3500 and 4500g and increases again beyond 4500g (*see* Chapters 1 and 2). Thus for populations of European origin the optimal range appears to lie between 3500 and 4500g. For populations such as those in Japan and China with a different pattern of birthweight distribution[1] the optimal range is likely to be lower.

In population terms, although the small number of infants born $<$ 2500g either due to preterm birth or intrauterine growth retardation are at greatly increased risk, as Power[2] points out 'when the risk is diffused throughout the population a large proportion of the population affected by a small risk may have a greater impact on population levels of disease than a smaller proportion at high risk' (p. 1270). To illustrate this point, data from West Sussex are shown again (*see* Table 7.1 and also Table 1.3, Chapter 1).

Table 7.1: Cerebral palsy prevalence by birthweight group in West Sussex, 1982–96

Birthweight group	Cerebral palsy	Without cerebral palsy	Rate/1000
< 1500g (n = 849)	55	794	64.7
1500–1999g (n = 1386)	37	1349	26.6
2000–2499g (n = 4192)	34	4158	8.1
2500–2999g (n = 16 942)	49	16 893	2.9
3000–3499g (n = 39 143)	60	39 083	1.5
3500–3999g (n = 31 692)	43	31 649	1.3
4000–4499g (n = 9939)	10	9929	1.0
≥ 4500g (n = 1559)	4	1555	2.6

The table shows that, despite the very high rates of cerebral palsy among infants born < 1500g, almost as many cases are contributed to the total by infants born between 2500–2999g and more by those born between 3000–3499g.[3]

Among populations of European origin, those with larger proportions of births in the optimal range tend to have lower rates of infant mortality (IMR) and vice versa (*see* Chapter 3, Table 3.3).[4] Norway and Sweden with 49.0% and 50.5% of births in the sub-optimal range (< 3500g) had low IMRs in the 1970s compared with the UK with 64.8% in the sub-optimal range and Hungary with 73.1%.[4]

In summary, the objective of promoting birthweight within an optimal range in a population shifts the focus to the whole birthweight distribution rather than just the lower extremes taking account of changes in distribution within the traditional 'normal' birthweight range (≥ 2500g) that are likely to significantly affect health outcomes across the lifecourse.

Why have interventions aimed at preventing low birthweight and preterm birth had limited success?

As already discussed in Chapters 4 and 5, systematic reviews of controlled trials of nutritional, antenatal care and social support interventions in the index pregnancy show little positive effect on either intrauterine growth or gestational duration particularly in developed countries.[5-7] Similar disappointing results have been reported with interventions designed to prevent preterm birth by treating bacterial vaginosis[8] and asymptomatic bacteriuria[9] in pregnancy and even prevention programmes combining a range of different interventions have had limited impact on pregnancy outcomes.[10]

A major limitation of many prevention programmes and interventions is that they are confined to the index pregnancy. As has been shown in Chapter 6, many of the determinants of intrauterine growth and gestational duration have their origins long before pregnancy. Some, such as maternal height and pre-pregnancy weight, are clearly not modifiable once pregnancy is established and others, such as smoking, chronic stress and lack of social support, tend to be well-established long before pregnancy and are more difficult to modify in the short period between pregnancy recognition and pregnancy outcome. Even those conditions, such as pregnancy-induced hypertension (PIH) and genital vaginosis, for which specific therapeutic interventions are available, have social and behavioural precursors stretching back into childhood and adolescence.

Pregnancy tends to be professionally confirmed between 10–20 weeks with the highest risk groups tending towards the upper limit of the range. Consequently, preventive programmes confined to the index pregnancy have a limited period in which to modify the limited number of risk factors that are theoretically open to modification. Risk factors, for example micronutrient deficiencies such as folate, may already have had an adverse impact on pregnancy during the first trimester prior to professional recognition. Even culturally sensitive interventions designed to reduce stress may be started too late in pregnancy to have any realistic chance of impacting on chronic stress.[11]

The tendency for preventive programmes to focus on the lower extremes of the birthweight and gestational age distribution may also contribute to the apparent lack of success associated with these interventions. Many report only effects on preterm birth or low birthweight without reference to potentially significant changes in the remainder of the birthweight distribution. The narrow definition of adverse pregnancy outcomes to include only those associated with the highest risk of adverse neonatal outcomes may mask shifts in the birthweight distribution attributable to the intervention.

With a few notable exceptions such as those multi-factor intervention programmes reviewed by Alexander *et al.*,[10] most interventions have been designed to address a single, theoretically modifiable risk factor. Weight gain during pregnancy, smoking in pregnancy, genital and urinary infections, PIH, and lack of social support are some examples of single risk factors for which interventions have been designed and tested (*see* Chapters 4 and 5). The complex interplay of risk factors in the determination of pregnancy outcomes illustrated in Chapter 6 highlights the limitations of single risk factor approaches. For example, smoking in pregnancy cessation programmes, although demonstrating some positive effects on smoking rates,[12] are limited by the strong association of smoking in pregnancy with social disadvantage in developed countries[13] leading to poor uptake of programmes and higher attrition rates among disadvantaged smokers and socially patterned quit rates in cessation programmes.[14]

Many intervention studies have concentrated only on those at high risk of adverse pregnancy outcome. It may be that this high risk strategy when trying to prevent multi-factorial outcomes such as low birthweight or preterm birth is theoretically less likely to be successful than a universal strategy aimed at all pregnancies. As with the overwhelming majority of 'diseases' and conditions open to preventive interventions, low birthweight and preterm birth are part of a process or continuum rather than dichotomous states of 'disease' versus normality.[15] The cut-off points used to define these 'abnormal states' are arbitrary and do not delineate abnormality from normality. In such situations, interventions directed at high risk groups are subject to the following weaknesses identified by Rose:[15]

- Prevention becomes medicalised transforming women coming to pregnancy who thought they were normal into patients with consequences for the development of anxiety.
- The high risk approach does not seek to alter the situations which determine exposure nor to attack the underlying reasons why preterm birth and low birthweight exist – it simply offers protection to the most vulnerable individuals from the effects of a hazardous situation which is allowed to continue.
- Interventions requiring behavioural change on the part of individuals (for example smoking cessation in pregnancy) are likely to be particularly difficult for high risk individuals to do because it involves stepping out of line with the behaviour of their families and friends. In other words, health-related behaviours are not simply a matter of individual choice but are moulded and conditioned by societal norms and the behaviour of family and friends.
- Although high risk strategies are able to identify groups of women with higher levels of risk of adverse pregnancy outcome, they are very poor predictors of outcome for individual women within the group.
- The contribution to overall control of adverse pregnancy outcomes may be disappointingly small because risk is not confined to a small and readily identified segment of pregnant women and the efficacy of a high risk strategy in modifying risk across a whole population will depend on the ways in which risk and exposure are distributed throughout the population.

Kramer *et al.*[16] are correct to point out that 'it is the individuals within a society who are exposed to its socio-economic conditions and whose reactions and responses to those conditions alter their risk of adverse pregnancy outcome' (p. 197). However, the socio-economic and other factors bearing on individual women coming to pregnancy in different societies are determined not by the risk profiles of the individual women but by the social and health policies of those societies. Major differences in pregnancy outcomes have been noted between populations of European origin (i.e. relatively genetically homogeneous),[17] despite the similarity of risk factors affecting pregnancy outcomes, suggesting that policy differences at societal level may be important. It is possible that societal level determinants exert an influence on pregnancy outcomes such that individual level changes are unlikely to happen without significant societal level change thus imposing limitations on preventive approaches at the individual level. The potential effect of societal level of determinants has received little or no attention in the literature related to prevention of adverse pregnancy outcomes and, although there is reason to believe that societal level interventions could have a profound effect on pregnancy outcomes, further research is needed to test this belief (*see* Chapter 8).

Why have interventions aimed at preventing low birthweight and preterm birth had limited success?

- Interventions have been directed almost exclusively at the index pregnancy.
- For the small number of modifiable risk factors occurring in the index pregnancy, the time period available for effective intervention is short particularly amongst the more disadvantaged groups who tend to have their pregnancies professionally identified late.
- Limitation of the outcome to the lower extremes of the birthweight distribution may mask significant changes elsewhere in the birthweight distribution.
- The complex interplay of risk exposures contributing to adverse pregnancy outcomes is likely to result in limited results for interventions directed at single risk exposures.
- There are strong theoretical reasons why preventive strategies directed at high risk groups are unlikely to have a major impact on the distribution of birthweight and/or gestational duration within a population.
- Interventions at the individual level may be ineffective if societal level determinants of adverse pregnancy outcomes have a strong limiting effect on risk exposures at the individual level.

Extending the biopsychosocial model to include societal level influences

As pointed out above, it is individual women in a population with their own characteristics who experience pregnancy and through whom the biological effects of social conditions are transmitted. However, the characteristics of those women such as their SES, education level, and nutritional status are strongly influenced by factors operating at the societal level beyond the control of the individual. For many women in developing countries the societal constraints on their social, educational and nutritional status allow little or no room for individual choice or social mobility. Although women in developed countries have more room for individual choice, societal factors continue to play a significant role in determining social, educational and nutritional status throughout the lifecourse.

Extending the model poses particular problems because of the relative lack of empirical data directly linking societal factors with the variables shown in the individual level model (*see* Figure 6.11, p. 140). Some associations of societal level with individual level factors are self-evident. For example, the ethnicity of individuals within a population is self-evidently associated with the history of migration into that population and its consequent ethnic composition. Empirical evidence linking societal level with the individual level characteristics depicted in the individual level model (*see* Figure 6.11, p. 140) is briefly reviewed to inform the extension of the model to include societal level influences.

Societal influences on SES at the individual level

In all countries SES varies across the population, although the extent of the variation can change, and this is reflected in marked differences in SES among women at the time of their birth and when they come to pregnancy. However, distribution of SES varies between countries and populations. Developing countries tend to have social distributions weighted heavily towards the lower end of the distribution with a very high proportion of their population living in absolute poverty. Richer developed countries have smaller proportions of their populations in the lower tail of the distribution but distributions vary considerably even between rich countries with similar levels of wealth.[18]

The distribution of SES across populations is influenced by the overall wealth of the country and income distribution and the level of tax and credit transfer.[19] Among rich industrial nations in the late 1990s, rates of child poverty (% of families with children with incomes < 50% of the national median income) varied from 2.6% in Sweden to 19.8% the UK and 22.4% in the USA.[20]

Differences in SES distribution among families with children between countries with similar per capita levels of gross domestic product are partly explained by differences in tax and credit transfer.[20] For example, Sweden in 1991 converted a 'market child poverty rate' (proportion of families with children in poverty before tax and credit transfer) among lone parent families from 40% to < 5% after tax and credit transfer.[21] In contrast, the USA in 1991 only managed to reduce 'market child poverty' among lone parent families from 60% to 50%

after income transfers.[21] Two other major associated economic factors determine differences in child poverty rates: the proportion of households with children in which no adult is working and the proportion of households with children headed by an adult earning less than two-thirds of the national median income.[20] In developing countries, more equitable income distribution can offset the impact of poverty on children and families.[22]

The link between income distribution, tax and employment policy and individual level SES is supported by the above evidence. Income distribution and employment are influenced by national and global economic policies and trends and can change dramatically over relatively short periods. For example, income inequalities in the UK increased sharply during the 1980s associated with a threefold increase in child poverty rates.[23] Unemployment increased especially among families with young children resulting in 19.1% of households with children having no adult in work in 1996 falling again to 15.3% in 2001.[23] Thus, the model needs to reflect potential changes in these economic indicators over the woman's life course from infancy to pregnancy.

Income distribution and tax policy also influence levels of child and maternity benefits. These benefits, designed to offset some of the excess cost associated with pregnancy and child rearing, are universal in many European countries but levels vary. The UK has one of the lowest levels of maternity and child benefits among comparable European countries.

Societal level influences on individual educational attainment

Education is closely linked to SES and is often used as a measure of SES.[22] Kramer et al.[16] identified education as 'the dimension of SES that most strongly and consistently predicts health, especially for women and children' (p. 196). Although individual women have individual education levels measurable as years of education or qualifications obtained, their educational attainment is dependent on the availability and accessibility of education at a societal level. Women living in developing countries where education is either not provided or access is difficult for geographical, economic or cultural reasons are likely to have low levels of education for societal rather than individual reasons. Developed countries tend to have universal access to education for girls as well as boys with literacy levels approaching 100%. However, in a similar way to income, distribution of educational attainment varies between rich nations.[24] Figure 7.1 shows the distribution of document literacy (knowledge and skills required to locate and use information contained in various formats) and prose literacy (knowledge and skills needed to understand and use information from texts including editorials, instruction manuals etc.) levels among people aged 16–65 across Organization of Economic Cooperation & Development (OECD) countries participating in the International Adult Literacy Study.[24] Sweden has more than 70% of its population with document and prose literacy at the higher levels (levels 3, 4 and 5) and a very small percentage at level 1. By contrast, in the UK and the USA, although 50% of the population are at levels 3, 4 and 5, approximately 20% are at the lowest level (level 1) for both types of literacy.

The OECD study also shows a close correlation between income distribution and educational attainment such that the more unequal the income distribution the more unequal the levels of educational attainment across the social strata (*see* Figure 7.2).[24] As a result of inequalities in the distribution of educational attainment, the UK and the USA have relatively large proportions of sub-literacy and sub-numeracy among their adult populations.

Intelligence at five years of age, as measured by IQ, and maths ability aged seven to eight years and nine to ten years have been shown in the US National Longitudinal Study of Youth (Child Supplement) to demonstrate a stepwise graded association with income-to-needs ratios such that there was a greater than 16 point difference in IQ at five years between those children in deep poverty (income-to-needs ratio $\leqslant 0.5$) and those in affluent families (income-to-needs ratio $\geqslant 3$).[25] A similar gradient was reported for maths ability at ages seven to eight years and nine to ten years and the study suggests that these differences increase with increasing age.[25] These findings are consistent with those of the OECD study[24] as the more unequal the income distribution, the greater the number of children in poverty.

Thus, the distribution of literacy and numeracy, themselves influenced by income distribution, are included in the extended model (*see* Figure 7.3, p. 162) as societal influences on individual levels of educational attainment.

Societal influences on individual nutritional status

Nutritional status seems to exert its most important influence on pregnancy outcome through maternal height and weight at the onset of pregnancy (*see* Chapters 4 and 5). Height attained at seven years of age is strongly predict-ive of attained adult height[26] suggesting that nutritional influences in early childhood are a key environmental component of pre-pregnancy height. In pregnancy itself, extreme calorie deprivation, particularly in the third trimester, is known to be associated with impaired fetal growth[27] but, as discussed in Chapter 5, protein/energy supplementation in generally well-nourished popu-lations has not been shown in clinical trials to significantly increase birth-weight.[28] Although observational studies suggest a significant role for micronutrient deficiency in pregnancy outcomes, controlled trials of supplementation have reported little or no effect (*see* Chapter 5).[29]

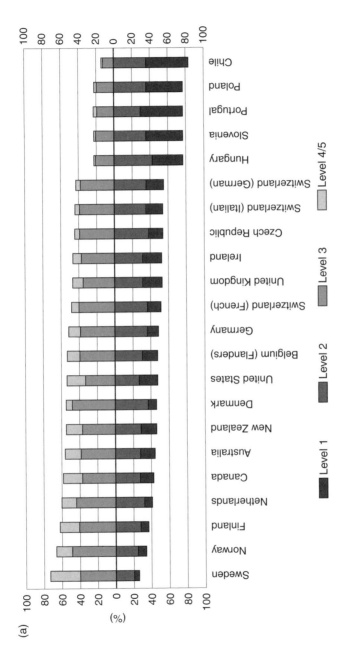

Figure 7.1a: Comparative distribution of literacy levels: percentage of population aged 16–65 at each literacy level; 1994–98: (a) prose literacy; (b) document literacy (countries ranked by the proportion in levels 3 and 4/5).

Source: OECD, p. 17.[24]

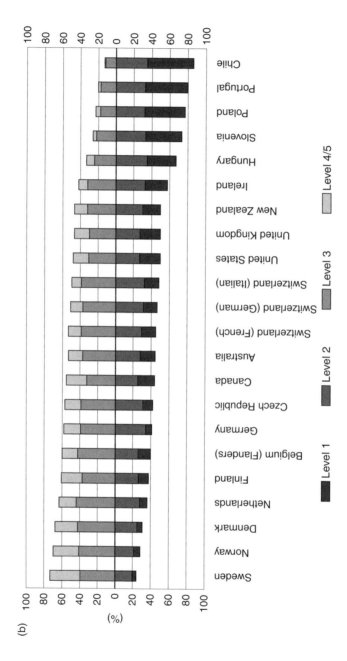

Figure 7.1b: *Continued*

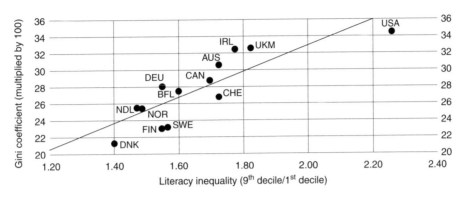

Figure 7.2: Relationship between income inequality (Gini coefficient) and inequality in the distribution of literacy (9th decile/1st decile) within countries, prose scale.

Food availability is a self-evident societal level influence on individual nutritional status in childhood and in pregnancy. Women living in societies subject to famine and food scarcity are likely to be undernourished simply because appropriate food is not available. In developed countries with abundant food sources, availability is related to cost and distribution policies employed by food manufacturers and retailers.[30] For example, in the UK, there is evidence that access to fruit and vegetables is more difficult for those living in poor areas without their own transport because 70% of fruit and vegetable sales are now made through supermarket chains whose shops are difficult to access without a car.[31] Healthier foods tend to be more expensive[30] and, even where supermarkets exist within poor areas, food has been shown to be more expensive than in more affluent areas.[32]

Among pregnant women in Avon, south-west England, those who stated that they had the greatest difficulty affording basic items, such as food, clothing, housing, and heating, had the worst diets.[33] This finding is consistent with other UK studies that have shown very low intakes of many nutrients especially iron, vitamins A and C, and folic acid among low income pregnant women.[34,35]

At a societal level, food availability, cost and differential distribution influence individual nutritional status. Societies with higher numbers of low income families resulting from greater income inequality are likely to have higher numbers of children experiencing poor nutrition in early childhood leading to stunting and higher numbers of women with low intakes of essential nutrients during pregnancy. Levels of child and maternity benefit and food entitlements during childhood and pregnancy are likely to be important in offsetting some of the adverse effects of poor nutritional status. Thus, food availability, cost, and distribution themselves influenced by income distribution and benefit levels are included in the extended model (*see* Figure 7.3, p. 162).

Societal influences on stress and psychological factors at the individual level

The relationship between stress and adverse psychological factors and socio-economic status has already been discussed in Chapter 6. Extrapolating from the individual to the societal level, it seems reasonable to assume that, in a society with higher levels of relative poverty, a higher proportion of women would be exposed to stressful situations and depression. Although there is little direct empirical evidence to support this assumption, there is a considerable body of work suggesting that high levels of income inequality among developed countries are associated with adverse health outcomes[18] partly through mechanisms related to reduced social coherence in more unequal societies. Social coherence, itself influenced by income distribution, is included in the extended model (*see* Figure 7.3, p. 162).

Societal influences on maternal age and parity

The association of maternal age and parity at the individual level is discussed in Chapter 6. As Table 7.2 shows, the 1998 teenage birth rates among 25 developed countries are correlated with income distribution represented by the Gini coefficient. The moderate correlation ($r = 0.44$) suggests that countries with higher levels of income inequality tend to have higher levels of teenage pregnancy known to be associated with negative pregnancy outcomes (*see* Chapter 5).

The UNICEF report[36] based on 28 of the world's wealthiest countries states that societies that were successful in preparing their young people to cope with a more sexualised society as well as those still committed to more traditional family values were more likely to have lower levels of teenage pregnancy. The influence of income distribution on maternal age is included in the extended model (*see* Figure 7.3, p. 162).

Societal influences on antenatal care availability and utilisation

Although available evidence suggests a limited role for antenatal care in the prevention of preterm delivery and low birthweight (*see* Chapter 5), it is clear that interventions related to infection and pregnancy-induced hyptertension in the index pregnancy can be instituted only if antenatal care is available, accessible and utilised by pregnant women. In countries in which antenatal services are not available, these medical problems cannot be treated. Among

Table 7.2: Teenage pregnancy rates 1998 in OECD countries by Gini coefficient

Country	Teenage birth rate 1998	Gini coefficient (×100) 1998
Switzerland	5.5	35.5
Netherlands	6.2	30.2
Sweden	6.5	25.3
Italy	6.6	35.9
Spain	7.9	32.4
Denmark	8.1	24.6
Belgium	9.9	27.7
Finland	9.2	24.6
France	9.3	32.4
Luxembourg	9.7	26.9
Greece	11.8	35.6
Germany	13.1	30.0
Norway	12.4	25.7
Austria	14.0	30.4
Czech Republic	16.4	25.8
Ireland	18.7	34.6
Australia	18.4	33.7
Poland	18.7	35.8
Portugal	21.2	38.2
Hungary	26.5	25.0
Slovak Republic	26.9	26.2
New Zealand	29.8	37.0
UK	30.8	36.6
Canada	20.2	31.7
USA	52.1	40.6

Pearson correlation r = 0.44 (p < 0.05).

Source: UNICEF, p. 15.[36]

countries with well-developed antenatal services, cost may prevent poor women from accessing adequate levels of antenatal care. In the USA, for example, 43.1 million people were uninsured in 1997[37] severely limiting their access to adequate health services. Even in countries such as the UK with 'free-at-the-time-of-use' health services, utilisation of antenatal services is socially patterned with women in lower social groups less likely to book for antenatal care early and less likely to attend so frequently.[38] Antenatal care availability and cost are included in the extended model (*see* Figure 7.3, p. 162) as they affect the management and treatment of pregnancy complications such as vaginosis and PIH.

The extended biopsychosocial model

The extended model incorporating the societal influences on individual level factors determining birthweight is shown in Figure 7.3.

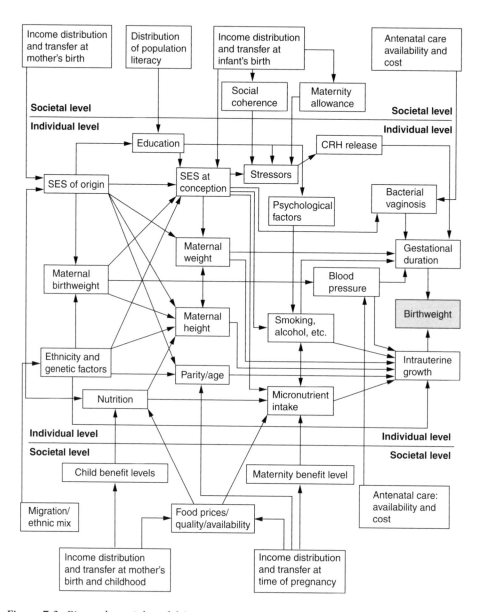

Figure 7.3: Biopsychosocial model 2.

> **Societal level influences on individual level determinants of pregnancy outcome**
>
> - There is strong evidence linking societal level factors to individual level SES, educational status, nutritional status, age at pregnancy and antenatal care availability and utilisation.
> - Combined with individual level determinants, these societal influences form the basis for an extended explanatory model of birthweight determination.

Alternative approaches to promoting optimal birthweight based on the extended biopsychosocial model

As the extended version of the model shows (*see* Figure 7.3), many of the risk exposures of importance at the individual level before and during pregnancy are strongly influenced by societal level determinants. However, health professionals and the services in which they work deal with individual women before and during pregnancy and it is possible that most benefit will accrue from promotional strategies directed at both individual and societal levels. Time scales also play a part in considering strategies: societal level change is likely to have its effect in the long term; individual level change may also require more long-term approaches but promotional approaches cannot simply ignore women coming to pregnancy in the short and medium term. Thus, alternative strategies need to combine effective individual and societal level interventions operating within the short, medium and long term.

Buekens and Klebanoff[39] acknowledge the need for alternative approaches to prevention because of the failure of interventions to decrease the rate of preterm birth. They identify the change of emphasis towards the links between social and biological mechanisms including the impact on stress of racism and poverty and gene-environment interactions, and the need to explore the impact of broad contextual factors, such as universal social protection on preterm birth. Promotion of optimal birthweight, including prevention of preterm birth, will require a similar change of emphasis. The approaches discussed below should not be considered in isolation but combined to take account of the cumulative, additive and intergenerational effects as well as the societal and individual influences shown in the extended model (*see* Figure 7.3). Combining these approaches will require population-wide strategies with the objective of improving what Baird[40] calls 'the reproductive efficiency' of the women of childbearing age. The social and health policy implications of population-wide strategies are considered in the final chapter (*see* Chapter 8).

Interventions in pregnancy (short-term) that are likely to contribute positively to population-wide strategies to promote optimal birthweight

- Antenatal care that is culturally and socially sensitive, affordable by the poorest groups in society, readily accessible to all women, and flexible enough to cover particular high-risk groups such as adolescent mothers.
- Maternity benefits and income transfer sufficient to ensure that no pregnant woman is prevented by cost from consuming a diet containing sufficient levels of recommended nutrients. Further research is needed to establish an adequate income level to fulfill this requirement in each country (*see* Chapter 8). This was a key recommendation of the Independent Inquiry into Inequalities in Health in the UK (the Acheson Report) published in 1998.[41]
- Measures to reduce food poverty and increase the availability and accessibility of foodstuffs to supply an adequate and affordable diet for all sections of the population will help to ensure that pregnant mothers are less likely to experience difficulty consuming an adequate diet (also recommended in the Acheson Report).[41]
- Measures to alleviate chronic stress and buffer its effects including the financial measures considered above and community-level interventions offering assistance to women that they themselves perceive as socially supportive. More research is needed in this area (*see* Chapter 8) but there is some indication from a study among low income black women in the USA that social support tailored to the needs of the women in the population is associated with an increase in birthweight.[42] Further research is needed to confirm the effectiveness of social support interventions tailored to the expressed needs of pregnant women (*see* Chapter 8).
- Smoking cessation programmes have been shown to be effective during pregnancy[12] but uptake tends to be poorer and drop-out rates higher among those most likely to smoke.[14] Given the association of smoking both with stress[43] and low income,[13] smoking rates may reduce if the interventions related to income and stress are instituted. It is also possible that smoking cessation programmes sensitive to social context[44] might be associated with higher participation and lower attrition rates among low income women.

Interventions in childhood, adolescence and prior to pregnancy (medium- and long-term) that are likely to contribute positively to population-wide strategies to promote optimal birthweight

- Measures to reduce levels of child poverty and ensure that children have access to sufficient income to participate fully in the society in which they live. Recent work on child poverty in Britain[45] suggests that 41% of lone parent families with one child, 54% of lone parents with two children and 15% of couples with one child live on incomes insufficient to 'make ends meet' (defined by the researchers as 'absolute' poverty). The weekly income, after tax, said to be needed to avoid 'absolute' poverty averages £178 for all types of households (p. 55).[45] A Canadian study[46] attempts to define an income level below which children's health is seriously compromised. As indicated above, rich countries that have succeeded in reducing child poverty levels have done so by effective tax and credit transfer and greater equality of income distribution.[20] Social and economic policies required to reduce child poverty are discussed in more detail in Chapter 8.
- Measures to improve the educational status of all children in the population and reduce levels of sub-literacy and sub-numeracy. Societal influences on individual educational attainment and the importance of educational attainment to pregnancy outcome have been considered above.
- Measures to ensure affordable and high quality early childcare and education available to all. Attempts in the UK to encourage mothers with young children to work have been hampered by lack of affordable childcare.[47] Of equal importance is the potential importance of high quality early childhood education in ensuring school readiness and enabling children to benefit fully from education.[48,49]
- Measures to reduce food poverty and increase the availability and accessibility of foodstuffs to supply an adequate and affordable diet for all sections of the population will help to ensure that young girls' growth is optimised before the age of seven years.
- Measures to provide accessible and readily available contraceptive services for young people combined with appropriate and open sex education as part of a strategy to reduce teenage pregnancies in some rich nations such as the UK and the USA. As discussed above, income distribution appears to be closely correlated to teenage pregnancy rates but availability of affordable contraceptive services and non-judgmental sex education appear to provide further protection to young people.[36]

- Measures to reduce teenage uptake of smoking and to increase quit rates particularly amongst young women. Health education has not proved effective alone in promoting non-smoking. The Acheson Report[41] recommends measures aimed at restricting smoking in public places, abolishing smoking advertising and promotion, and price increases to discourage young people from becoming habitual smokers.

References

1 Evans S and Alberman E (1989) International Collaborative Effort (ICE) on birthweight; plurality; and perinatal and infant mortality: II. Comparisons between birthweight distributions of births in member countries from 1970 to 1984. *Acta Obstetr Gynaecol Scand.* **68**: 11–7.

2 Power C (1994) National trends in birth weight: implications for future adult disease. *BMJ.* **308**: 1270–1.

3 Sundrum R, Logan S, Wallace A and Spencer NJ (2002) (submitted for publication).

4 Saugstad LF (1981) Weight of all births and infant mortality. *J Epidemiol and Comm Health.* **35**: 185–91.

5 Kramer MS (1998) Balanced protein/energy supplementation in pregnancy (Cochrane Review). In: The Cochrane Library (Issue 4). Update Software, Oxford.

6 Kramer MS (1987) Determinants of low birth weight: methodological assessment and meta-analysis. *Bull WHO.* **65**: 663–737.

7 Hodnett ED (2000) Support during pregnancy for women at increased risk (Cochrane Review). In: The Cochrane Library (Issue 1). Update Software, Oxford.

8 Brocklehurst P, Hannah M and McDonald H (1998) The management of bacterial vaginosis in pregnancy (Cochrane Review). In: The Cochrane Library (Issue 4), Update Software, Oxford.

9 Smaill F (1998) Antibiotics vs. no treatment for asymptomatic bacteriuria in pregnancy (Cochrane Review). In: Cochrane Library (Issue 4). Update Software, Oxford.

10 Alexander GS, Weiss J, Hulsey TC and Papiernik E (1991) Preterm birth prevention: an evaluation of programs in the United States. *Birth.* **18**: 160–9.

11 Manaseki S, Spencer NJ, Aveyard P and Forster D (2002) A systematic review of randomised controlled trials of the provision of social support to reduce preterm delivery. The case for more rigorous RCTs. (submitted for publication).

12 Lumley J, Oliver S and Waters E (2001) Interventions for promoting smoking cessation during pregnancy (Cochrane Review). In: The Cochrane Library (Issue 3). Update Software, Oxford.

13 Graham H (1996) Smoking prevalence among women in the European Community, 1950 to 1990. *Soc Sci and Med.* **43**: 243–54.

14 Dolan-Mullen P (1999) Maternal smoking during pregnancy and evidence based interventions to promote cessation. *Primary Care.* **26**: 577–89.

15 Rose G (1992) *The Strategy of Preventive Medicine.* Oxford Medical Publications, Oxford.

16 Kramer MS, Séguin L, Lydon J and Goulet L (2000) Socio-economic disparities in pregnancy outcome: why do the poor fare so poorly? *Paed and Perinatal Epidemiol.* **14**: 194–210.

17 Koupilová I, Vågerö D, Leon DA, Pikhart H *et al.* (1998) Social variation in size at birth and preterm delivery in the Czech Republic and Sweden, 1989–91. *Paed and Perinatal Epidemiol.* **12**: 7–24.

18 Wilkinson RG (1996) *Unhealthy Societies: the afflictions of inequality.* Routledge, London.

19 Smeeding TS, O'Higgins M, Rainwater L and Atkinson AB (1990) *Poverty, Inequality and Income Distribution in Comparative Perspective.* Simon Schuster, London.

20 UNICEF (2000) *A League Table of Child Poverty in Rich Nations.* Innocenti Research Report No 2, UNICEF Innocenti Research Centre, Florence.

21 Ross DP, Scott K and Kelly M (1996) *Child Poverty: what are the consequences?* Centre for International Statistics, Canadian Council on Social Development, Ottawa, Canada.

22 Spencer NJ (2000) *Poverty and Child Health* (2e). Radcliffe Medical Press, Oxford: pp. 100–32.

23 Howard M, Garnham A, Fimister G and Viet-Wilson J (2001) *Poverty: the facts* (4e). Child Poverty Action Group, London.

24 Organization of Economic Cooperation & Development (OECD) (2001) *Literacy in the Information Age.* OECD, Paris.

25 Brooks-Gunn J, Duncan G and Britto PB (1999) Are socioeconomic gradients for children similar to those for adults? Achievement and health of children in the United States. In: DP Keating and C Hertzman (eds) *Developmental Health and the Wealth of Nations.* The Guilford Press, New York and London: pp. 94–124.

26 Power C, Manor O and Fox J (1991) *Health and Class: the early years.* Chapman & Hall, London.

27 Susser M and Stein Z (1994) Timing in prenatal nutrition: a reprise of the Dutch famine study. *Nutrition Rev.* **52**: 84–94.

28 Kramer MS (1998) Balanced protein/energy supplementation in pregnancy (Cochrane Review). In: The Cochrane Library (Issue 4). Update Software, Oxford.

29 Ramakrishnan U, Manjrekar R, Rivera J, Gonzáles-Cossío T and Martorell R (1999) Micronutrients and pregnancy outcome: a review of the literature. *Nutrition Res.* **19**: 103–59.

30 Dowler E, Turner S and Dobson B (2001) *Poverty Bites: food, health and poor families.* Child Poverty Action Group, London.

31 Dowler E, Blair D, Rex A, Donkin A and Grundy C (2001) *Mapping Access to Healthy Food in Sandwell.* Report to the Sandwell Health Action Zone, Sandwell.

32 Sooman A, Macintyre S and Anderson A (1993) Scotland's health – a more difficult challenge for some? The price and availability of healthy foods in socially contrasting localities in the West of Scotland. *Health Bull.* **51**: 276–84.

33 Rogers I, Emmett P, Baker D, Golding J and the ALSPAC study team (1998) Financial difficulties, smoking habits, composition of diet and birthweight in a population of pregnant women in the South West of England. *Eur J Clin Nutrition.* **52**: 251–60.

34 Schofield C, Stewart J and Wheeler E (1989) The diets of pregnant and post-pregnant women in different social groups in London and Edinburgh: calcium, iron, retinol, ascorbic acid, and folic acid. *Br J Nutrition.* **62**: 363–77.

35 Dallison J and Lobstein T (1995) *Poor Expectations: poverty and undernourishment in pregnancy.* NCH Action for Children and the Maternity Alliance, London.

36 UNICEF (2001) *A League Table of Teenage Births in Rich Nations.* Innocenti Report Card No 3, UNICEF Innocenti Research Centre, Florence.

37 Lillie-Blanton M, Martinez RM, Lyons B and Rowland D (1999) *Access to Health Care: promises and prospects for low-income Americans.* The Kaiser Commission on Medicaid and the Uninsured, The Henry J Kaiser Family Foundation, Washington DC.

38 Cliff D and Deery R (1997) Too much like school: social class, age, marital status and attendance/non-attendance at antenatal classes. *Midwifery.* **13**: 139–45.

39 Buekens P and Klebanoff M (2001) Preterm birth research: from disillusion to the search for new mechanisms. *Paed and Perinatal Epidemiol.* **15** (Suppl 2): 159–61.

40 Baird D (1980) Environment and reproduction. *Br J Obstetr and Gynaecol.* **87**: 1057–67.

41 Department of Health (1998) *Independent Inquiry into Inequalities in Health:* The Acheson Report. The Stationery Office, London.

42 Norbeck JS, DeJoseph JF and Smith RT (1996) A randomized trial of an empirically-derived social support intervention to prevent low birth weight among African American women. *Soc Sci and Med.* **43**: 947–54.

43 Sheehan TJ (1998) Stress and low birth weight: a structural modeling approach using real life stressors. *Soc Sci and Med.* **47**: 1503–12.

44 Blackburn C and Graham H (1993) *Smoking Amongst Working Class Mothers – an information pack.* Department of Applied Social Studies, University of Warwick, Coventry.

45 Gordon D (2000) Measuring absolute and overall poverty. In: D Gordon and P Townsend (eds) *Breadline Europe: the measurement of poverty.* The Policy Press, Bristol.

46 Ross DP and Roberts P (1999) *Income and Child Well-being: a new perspective on the poverty debate.* Canadian Council on Social Development, Ottawa.

47 Law C (1999) Mother, fetus, infant, child and family: socio-economic inequalities. In: D Gordon, M Shaw, D Dorling and G Davey Smith (eds) *Inequalities in Health: evidence presented to the Independent Inquiry into Inequalities in Health, chaired by Sir Donald Acheson.* The Policy Press, Bristol.

48 Schweinhart LJ, Barnes HV and Weikart DP (1993) *Significant Benefits: the High/Scope Perry Preschool Study through age 27.* High/Scope Press, Ypsilanti.

49 Sylva K and Wilshire J (1993) The impact of early learning on children's later development: a review prepared for the RSA inquiry 'Start Right'. *Eur Early Childhood Education Res J.* **1**: 17–40.

CHAPTER 8

Implications of the biopsychosocial model for research, clinical practice and health policy

This chapter seeks to draw together the threads of the preceding chapters in order to recommend directions for research, clinical practice, and health and social policy consistent with the individual level (*see* Figure 6.11) and extended biopsychosocial models (*see* Figure 7.3) discussed in Chapters 6 and 7.

A core theme of the book has been the intimate relationship between biological and social factors influencing pregnancy outcome. Although pregnancy is clearly a biological process involving complex biological mechanisms and pathways, it takes place within individuals living within specific societies at particular periods of their historical and social development. Social exposures, in part determined by societal factors pertaining throughout the woman's life course, exert their influence on pregnancy outcome by modifying biological processes. Clinical practice alone, with its primary focus on biological processes, can have only a marginal effect on pregnancy outcome. As discussed in Chapter 7, strategies to promote optimal birthweight and pregnancy outcome need to encompass a range of short-, medium- and long-term measures consistent with the extended biopsychosocial model (*see* Figure 7.3, p. 162). In this chapter, the implications of the promotional strategies discussed in Chapter 7 for research, clinical practice and health policy are considered and future directions recommended.

The models derived in Chapters 6 and 7 are tentative, incomplete and theoretical. They have yet to be confirmed in empirical research. For this reason, this chapter starts by considering the research implications of the models and the directions needed to test and modify them in empirical data.

Clinical practice if not accompanied by social interventions may have a limited effect on pregnancy outcomes but it is an important medium through which short-term interventions to promote optimal birthweight can be directed. The implications of the biopsychosocial model for clinical practice are considered next.

Finally, health policies, incorporating social and economic policies, most likely to promote optimal birthweight in the short, medium and long term are considered. Based on the biopsychosocial models, it seems likely that health-promoting social and economic policies are essential if not sufficient for the promotion of optimal birthweight within populations.

Research directions in the promotion of optimal birthweight: implications of the biopsychosocial models

Exploring the mechanisms by which the social translates into the biological

Health-related research has tended to be divided into biological, psychological and social research with little attention to their inter-connections and inter-relationships. However, there is increasing interest in exploring the relationships and specifically the mechanisms by which biological processes are affected by social and psychological factors.[1,2] In pregnancy outcome research, the 'March of Dimes' research programme[3] is designed to test new ideas related to social and biological mechanisms and to generate new hypotheses. Kramer *et al.*'s study,[4] already discussed in Chapter 6, proposes to use path analysis to test a theoretical model of the determinants of social disparity in preterm birth. Their model (*see* Figure 6.10, p. 137) considers mechanisms by which social factors may influence biological processes: the possible effect of folate deficiency on gene expression; the possible effect of stress on corticotropin-releasing hormone (CRH) secretion. Rich-Edwards *et al.*[5] are studying women's experience of racism and violence and their potential effects on preterm birth through the mechanism of increased CRH secretion.

As I have argued in previous chapters, although preterm birth is the strongest determinant of low birthweight in developed countries, there is a powerful case for shifting the focus to sub-optimal birthweight. Studies of the translation of social, psychological, and environmental risks into biological mechanisms impacting on birthweight distribution as well as gestational duration are needed to enhance our understanding of the determination of sub-optimal birthweight. Such studies are essential to inform strategies to promote optimal birthweight in individual pregnancies and across populations.

The following are suggestions for studies to explore the mechanisms by which social, psychological and environmental risks impact on biological processes in pregnancy leading to sub-optimal birthweight:

- Secondary analysis of existing cohorts that have collected social, psychological and biological data throughout pregnancy. The Avon Longitudinal Study of Parents and Children[6] is a cohort study fulfilling these criteria.

- Secondary analysis of cohort studies with intergenerational data as well as social, psychological and biological data related to pregnancy. The 1958 British birth cohort[7] partially fulfils these criteria.
- Large population-based cohort studies designed to address specific research questions related to the pathways from social, psychological and environmental risk through biological processes to birthweight. Kramer *et al.*'s cohort[4] within which they are undertaking a nested case-control study could be used to study these processes and similar cohort studies could be established in other populations to explore similar issues.
- Observational studies suggest a possible relationship of stress with adverse pregnancy outcomes[8] but interventions designed to increase social support in pregnancy show little effect on birthweight or gestational duration.[9] However, further work is needed to develop interventions that have a proven impact on perceived social support and are tailored to the needs of the target population.[10] Clinical trials of these interventions would then be needed to test their effectiveness.
- Further observational studies on the relationship of biological markers of adverse pregnancy outcomes such as blood pressure, urinary tract infection and CRH with low SES in different populations.
- Studies to test and modify the theoretical model of birthweight determination at the individual level (*see* Figure 6.11).

Exploring the effect of societal level factors on risk at the individual level

Studies have reported differences in pregnancy outcomes by country (*see* Chapter 3) but few studies have explored the reasons for these differences.[11–13] Different definitions and data collection methods have made international comparisons problematic. However, such differences are surmountable and empirical data could be collected on the effect of social, economic and health policies on known risk factors for adverse pregnancy outcome. As with studies of the impact of social risk on biological factors, the outcome of interest should be the whole of the birthweight distribution rather than simply the lower tail. Buekens and Klebanoff[3] acknowledge the need to explore further the impact of what they call 'broad contextual factors' such as universal social protection, on preterm birth. This should be extended to consider the impact of these factors on birthweight across the distribution.

Whitehead *et al.*,[14] when discussing ways of researching the impact of public policy on inequalities in health, illustrate how societal influences may affect health outcomes across populations. They report a study of self-reported health among lone parents aged 16–65 in Britain and Sweden between 1979 and

1995. Although the risk of fair/poor health was the same for lone parents compared with couple parents in both countries, Figure 8.1 shows the higher prevalence rates of fair/poor health among British couple and lone parents compared with those in Sweden.

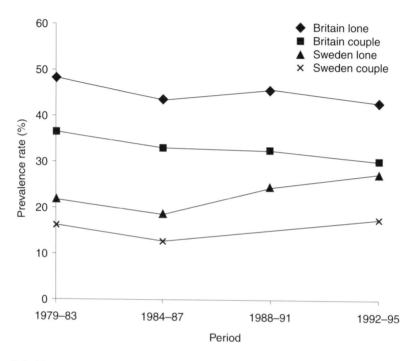

Figure 8.1: European standardised prevalence rates of less than good health, lone and couple mothers in Britain and in Sweden, ages 16–64, 1979–95.

Source: Whitehead *et al.*, p. 212.[14]

The authors suggest that specific policies, such as extensive, high quality, affordable daycare for children, family-friendly employment policies and adequate social security support, have protected Swedish parents, both couple and lone, from exposure to poverty and joblessness and thus protected their health. Although not directly relevant to the study of societal influences on pregnancy outcomes, this study illustrates both the possibility and value of studying these differences.

Some suggestions for studies to explore the effect of societal level factors on risk at the individual level are listed below:

- Studies of variation in risk exposures at the individual level between comparable countries and the extent of the variation explained by social and economic policy differences and migration histories.

- Studies comparing the population attributable risk (PAR) of exposures at the individual level in comparable countries and how these are related to societal level influences.
- Studies of the effects of societal factors such as tax and credit transfer, income distribution, and distribution of educational attainment on the intergenerational and life course experiences of cohorts of women (the methodology of Baird's study[12] could be modified and extended to include more countries).
- Studies of the effects of health service availability and accessibility in different countries on the management of biological risk factors during pregnancy.
- Studies of the relationship between birthweight distribution and gross national product and income distribution (Hales *et al.*[15] have demonstrated that national infant mortality rates are influenced by the distribution of income within societies: their method could be applied to birthweight).

Implications of the biopsychosocial models for clinical practice

Perhaps the most important message for clinical practice from the biopsychosocial models outlined in Chapters 6 and 7 is the limitations imposed on the effectiveness of clinical interventions in pregnancy in promoting optimal birthweight by the life course and intergenerational determinants of birthweight. Clinical interventions such as *in vitro* fertilisation and more sophisticated fetal monitoring appear to have pushed low birthweight rates up rather than promoting optimal birthweight.[16]

Despite these limitations, clinicians will continue to strive to ensure the optimal outcome for both mother and baby. The models suggest a need for clinicians to be sensitive to the social context in which the pregnancy is taking place and recognise the cumulative and additive effects of risk exposures. For example, smoking cessation advice offered in a judgmental way that fails to account for the social influences on smoking is likely to increase stress and be less likely to succeed in persuading the woman to quit smoking.

Clinicians have an important advocacy role informing politicians and policy makers of the value of promoting optimal birthweight and providing data on trends and determinants to support their advocacy. This is probably best done through national and local organisations of relevant and interested clinicians.

Implications of the biopsychosocial models for health and social policy

The models suggest that, whilst clinical interventions in the index pregnancy are of limited value in promoting optimal population levels of birthweight, health and social policy interventions in the short, medium and long term could be expected to have a profound effect on population birthweight distribution. The final part of Chapter 7 outlined interventions capable of promoting optimal birthweight and many of these are policy level interventions. These are discussed in more detail here. The interventions considered below broadly follow the recommendations of the Acheson Report[17] and, for this reason, tend to be most applicable to the UK although, in broad outline, they apply to any rich nation that has undergone the 'epidemiological transition'.[18] The overall objective of health and social policy aimed at promoting optimal birthweight should be to ensure that a high proportion of women come to, and go through, pregnancy in the best possible biological, psychological and social condition.

Poverty, income, tax and benefits

Reductions in levels of poverty and material deprivation among women of childbearing age and young children. There is likely to be a direct connection between the prevalence rates of poverty and material deprivation in a population and the proportion of women coming to pregnancy having experienced the adverse effects of material hardship in childhood and adolescence. Improving living standards of the poorest will require redistributive policies similar to those in place in Sweden and other Scandinavian countries (*see also* Chapter 7).[19] UNICEF estimate that the resources required to reduce child poverty in countries such as the UK form a small percentage of the gross national product.[20] Successfully reducing poverty and material deprivation among women of childbearing age and young children is likely to have short-, medium- and long-term effects on birthweight. In the short term, women are likely to be better nourished, experience less stress and smoke less at conception and during pregnancy. Smoking in pregnancy is very closely related to income levels[21] suggesting that increasing the income of women at the lowest income levels may have a direct effect on their chances of avoiding smoking in pregnancy. In the medium term, poverty reductions are likely to assist adolescent girls to avoid pregnancy and possibly influence their coping skills so that they are able to quit smoking prior to pregnancy. Teenage pregnancy,[22] coping[23] and quitting smoking prior to pregnancy[24] all appear to be sensitive to income levels. In the long term, policies to reduce the number of children living in material disadvantage and poverty are likely to be associated with improved levels of growth secondary to better nutrition and improved psychosocial development ensuring that a higher proportion of taller women who are less likely to suffer psychosocial problems come to pregnancy in the future. Growth,[25] cognitive[26] and psychosocial development[27] in early childhood are highly sensitive to material disadvantage and poverty.

Education

The development of universally available, affordable, high quality pre-school education enabling all children including the most disadvantaged to have access to educational interventions of proven value.[28] Early childhood is a critical and sensitive period in development and investment at this stage is likely to have the most benefit for the individual children and society.[29] As the biopsychosocial model suggests (*see* Figure 6.11), maternal education is a key variable in the determination of socio-economic status (SES) and psychosocial functioning and high quality pre-school education appears to be important in preparing children for school.[28] This policy will show benefits in the long term by ensuring that women come to pregnancy better educated and better prepared.

Educational policies designed to increase mean levels of literacy and numeracy among the adolescent and adult population and bring those at the lower end of the distribution up towards the mean. The aim should be to move the mean and distribution towards that of Sweden (*see* Figure 7.1, pp. 157–8).[30] The impact of these policies on birthweight is likely to be seen in the medium to long term.

Nutrition and food poverty

Policies to reduce food poverty and increase the availability and accessibility of foodstuffs to supply an adequate and affordable diet for all sections of the population but especially young children and women of child-bearing age. As Dowler *et al.*[31] suggest these policies will need to: ensure people have enough money for food, improve physical and economic access to food, support community food initiatives and local projects, protect mothers and babies and promote good food for children. These policies are likely to have short-, medium- and long-term effects on birthweight by improving nutrition during pregnancy, ensuring that women are well nourished at conception and reducing the prevalence of stunting among girls below the age of seven years so that fewer short women come to pregnancy in the future.

Sex education and contraceptive services for young people

Accessible and readily available contraceptive services for young people combined with appropriate and open sex education as part of a strategy to reduce teenage pregnancies to levels pertaining in the Netherlands and some other European countries. Combined with policies designed to redistribute income and reduce poverty (*see above*), freely available contraceptive services and non-judgmental sex education are likely to provide further protection to young people.[32] These policies are likely to have a medium-term impact on birthweight by ensuring that fewer immature young women come to pregnancy too early.

Smoking in pregnancy and among teenage girls

Policies to reduce teenage uptake of smoking and to increase quit rates particularly amongst young women. Health education has not proved effective alone in promoting non-smoking. The Acheson Report[17] recommends measures aimed at restricting smoking in public places, abolishing smoking advertising and promotion and price increases to discourage young people from becoming habitual smokers. Socially and culturally sensitive smoking cessation programmes in pregnancy, based on interventions of proven efficacy[33] modified to ensure participation by the most disadvantaged women, should be given priority especially in areas with high teenage and pregnancy smoking rates. These policies are likely to have a short-, medium- and long-term impact on birthweight by reducing the proportion of teenage girls who become established smokers and the proportion of women in the population smoking during pregnancy.

Antenatal care availability, affordability and accessibility

Despite the lack of evidence for the efficacy of antenatal services in promoting optimal birthweight (*see* Chapter 5), in the interests of equity and to ensure that smoking cessation and clinical interventions are available to all women independent of their area of residence or their financial resources, affordable, high quality antenatal services should be available to all women. Although the impact on birthweight may be small, effective health promotional, nutritional or clinical interventions may be developed in the future that can only be delivered to all women if they have access to high quality antenatal care.

Research, clinical and policy implications of the biopsychosocial models

- Observational studies with sub-optimal birthweight as the outcome at the individual level to test and modify the biopsychosocial model.
- Observational studies at the societal level to test and modify the extended model.
- Clinical practice sensitive to the social and cultural context of pregnancy and focused on promoting optimal birthweight.
- Health and social policies aimed at ensuring that the highest possible percentage of women come to, and go through, pregnancy in optimal biological, psychological and social conditions.

References

1 Brunner E (1996) The social and biological basis of cardiovascular disease in office workers. In: D Blane, E Brunner and R Wilkinson (eds) *Health and Social Organization*. Routledge, London and New York: pp. 272–99.

2 Coe CL (1999) Psychosocial factors and psychoneuroimmunology within a lifespan perspective. In: DP Keating and C Hertzman (eds) *Developmental Health and the Wealth of Nations: social, biological and educational dynamics*. Guilford Press, New York and London: pp. 201–19.

3 Buekens P and Klebanoff M (2001) Preterm birth research: from disillusion to the search for new mechanisms. *Paed and Perinatal Epidemiol*. **15** (Suppl 2): 159–61.

4 Kramer MS, Goulet L, Lydon J, Séguin L, McNamara H, Dassa C, Platt RW, Chen MF, Gauthier H, Genest J, Kahn S, Libman M, Rozen R, Masse R, Miner L, Asselin G, Benjamin A, Klein J and Koren G (2001) Socio-economic disparities in preterm birth: causal pathways and analysis. *Paed and Perinatal Epidemiol*. **15** (Suppl 2): 104–23.

5 Rich-Edwards J, Krieger N, Majzoub J, Zierler S, Lieberman E and Gillman M (2001) Maternal experiences of racism and violence as predictors of preterm birth: rationale and study design. *Paed and Perinatal Epidemiol*. **15** (Suppl 2): 124–35.

6 Golding J (1997) *ALSPAC – The Avon Longitudinal Study of Parents and Children: aims and study design*. ALSPAC protocol (4e). Institute of Child Health, Bristol.

7 Hennessy E, Alberman E (1998) Intergenerational influences affecting birth outcome: I. Birthweight for gestational age in the children of the 1958 British Birth Cohort. *Paed and Perinatal Epidemiol*. **12** (Suppl): 45–60.

8 Aveyard P, Forster D, Spencer NJ, Manaseki S, Fry-Smith A, Hyde C, Gardosi J and Cheng KK (2002) Does stress cause premature delivery? A systematic review of observational studies. *J Epidemiol and Comm Health* (in press).

9 Hodnett ED (2000) Support during pregnancy for women at increased risk (Cochrane Review). In: *The Cochrane Library* (Issue 1). Update Software, Oxford.

10 Manaseki S, Spencer NJ, Aveyard P and Forster D (2002) A systematic review of randomised controlled trials of the provision of social support to reduce preterm delivery. The case for more rigorous RCTs. (submitted for publication).

11 Erickson JD and Bjerkedal T (1982) Fetal and infant mortality in Norway and the United States. *JAMA*. **247**: 987–91.

12 Baird D (1980) Environment and reproduction. *Br J Obstetr and Gynaecol*. **87**: 1057–67.

13 Koupilová I, Vågerö D, Leon DA, Pikhart H *et al*. (1998) Social variation in size at birth and preterm delivery in the Czech Republic and Sweden, 1989–91. *Paed and Perinatal Epidemiol*. **12**: 7–24.

14 Whitehead M, Diderichsen F and Burström B (2000) Researching the impact of public policy on inequalities in health. In: H Graham (ed) *Understanding Health Inequalities*. Open University Press, Buckingham and Philadelphia: pp. 203–18.

15 Hales S, Howden-Chapman P, Salmond C, Woodward A and Mackenbach J (1999) National infant mortality rates in relation to gross national product and distribution of income. *Lancet*. **354**: 2047.

16 Daltveit AK, Vollset SE, Skjaerven R and Irgens LM (1999) Impact of multiple births and elective deliveries on the trends in low birth weight in Norway, 1967–1995. *Am J Epidemiol*. **149**: 1128–33.

17 Department of Health (1998) *Independent Inquiry into Inequalities in Health*: the Acheson Report. The Stationery Office, London.

18 Wilkinson RG (1996) *Unhealthy Societies: the afflictions of inequality*. Routledge, London: pp. 29–49.

19 Ross DP and Roberts P (1999) *Income and Child Well-being: a new perspective on the poverty debate*. Canadian Council on Social Development, Ottawa.

20 UNICEF (2000) *A League Table of Child Poverty in Rich Nations*. Innocenti Research Report No 2, UNICEF Innocenti Research Centre, Florence.

21 Graham H and Blackburn C (1998) The socio-economic patterning of health and smoking behaviour among mothers with young children on income support. *Sociol Health and Illness*. **20**: 215–40.

22 UNICEF (2001) *A League Table of Teenage Births in Rich Nations*. Innocenti Report Card No 3, UNICEF Innocenti Research Centre, Florence.

23 Power C and Hertzman C (1999) Health, well-being, and coping skills. In: D Keating and C Hertzman (eds) *Developmental Health and the Wealth of Nations*: Social, biological and educational dynamics. Guilford Press, New York and London: pp. 41–54.

24 White A, Freeth S and O'Brien M (1992) *Infant Feeding 1990*. HMSO, London.

25 Kuh D and Wadsworth M (1989) Parental height: childhood environment and subsequent adult height in a national birth cohort. *Int J Epidemiol*. **18**: 663–8.

26 Brooks-Gunn J, Duncan GJ and Britto PR (1999) Are socioeconomic gradients for children similar to those for adults? Achievement and health of children in the United States. In: DP Keating and C Hertzman (eds) *Developmental Health and the Wealth of Nations*: social, biological and educational dynamics. The Guilford Press, New York and London: pp. 94–124.

27 Sacker A, Schoon I and Bartley M (2002) Social inequality in educational achievement and psychosocial adjustment throughout childhood: magnitude and mechanisms. *Soc Sci and Med*. **55**: 863–80.

28 Sylva K and Wilshire J (1993) The impact of early learning on children's later development: a review prepared for the RSA inquiry 'Start Right'. *Eur Early Childhood Education Res J*. **1**: 17–40.

29 Keating D (1999) Developmental health as the wealth of nations. In: DP Keating and C Hertzman (eds) *Developmental Health and the Wealth of Nations: social, biological and educational dynamics*. Guilford Press, New York and London: pp. 337–47.

30 Organization of Economic Cooperation & Development (OECD) (2001) *Literacy in the Information Age*. OECD, Paris.

31 Dowler E, Turner S and Dobson B (2001) *Poverty Bites: food, health and poor families*. Child Poverty Action Group, London.

32 UNICEF (2001) *A League Table of Teenage Births in Rich Nations*. Innocenti Report Card No 3, UNICEF Innocenti Research Centre, Florence.

33 Dolan-Mullen P (1999) Maternal smoking during pregnancy and evidence based interventions to promote cessation. *Primary Care*. **26**: 577–89.

CHAPTER 9

Conclusions

This book has been written in an attempt to refocus the debate on the prevention of low birthweight and preterm birth that has tended to stall on the disappointing results of the evaluation of carefully designed preventive programmes (*see* Chapter 6). It has been driven by the conviction that fundamental improvements in mortality and morbidity in infancy, childhood and adulthood depend, in large part, on ensuring that fewer babies are born too early and/or too small and as many babies as possible achieve a birthweight within the optimal range. Populations that have high rates of low birthweight ($<$ 2500g) and preterm birth ($<$ 37 weeks' gestation) and a low proportion of infants born within the optimal birthweight range will have less healthy infants, children and adults. The book has been informed by an understanding that, although birthweight is the culmination of a biological process in individual women, social, environmental, cultural and psychological factors combine to directly or indirectly modify the biology. Despite imperfect knowledge of the precise mechanisms by which the social translates into the biological, there can be no doubt that birthweight results from a complex interplay of these influences acting between generations and over the woman's life course as well as within the pregnancy itself.

Clinicians strive to ensure the best pregnancy and neonatal outcomes and have had considerable success in reducing neonatal mortality despite the lack of change in rates of low birthweight or preterm birth; however, the desired changes at population level are more likely to come about as a result of political and economic initiatives. For this reason, the individual level biopsychosocial pathway model based on the complex interplay of intergenerational, life course and pregnancy influences has been extended to include the influence of societal factors on individual level risk exposures. This, in turn, has informed the research and health and social policy recommendations discussed in Chapter 8. The models on which the recommendations are based are not empirically tested and it could be regarded as an unsubstantiated leap of faith to move from them to policy recommendations. Further research is needed to test, modify and develop the models but, as I have argued in Chapter 7, there are good theoretical reasons for linking societal levels of risk exposure to population pregnancy outcomes. In addition, those societies that have pursued policy options similar to those outlined in Chapter 8 reducing societal levels of risk exposure have the best population pregnancy outcomes.

The main conclusions of the book are summarised below:

- Birthweight has major implications for survival, health, growth and cognitive development in infancy, childhood and into adult life – the optimal birthweight range for all these outcomes in European and African origin populations (and possibly others) is 3500–4500g (*see* Chapters 1 and 2).
- Birthweight has major public health implications and those European countries with the highest proportion of their births within this optimal range have the best neonatal and infant survival rates and are likely to have better levels of health, growth and cognitive function in childhood and adult life (*see* Chapter 3).
- There is a wealth of evidence that biological, social and environmental risk exposures impact on birthweight and gestational duration individually and in combination (*see* Chapters 4 and 5).
- Although further evidence is needed, there are indications that chronic stress among other psychological factors may impact on fetal growth and gestational duration (*see* Chapter 5).
- Risk factors for impaired fetal growth and reduced gestational duration tend to cluster cross-sectionally and accumulate longitudinally (*see* Chapter 6).
- Recognition of the temporal sequencing of risk exposures and the relationship of risk exposures to one another over the life course and across generations is essential to understanding the mechanisms by which birthweight is determined; variables need to be analysed as proximal and distal (*see* Chapter 6).
- A theoretical framework for a biopsychosocial model of birthweight determination should fulfil the following: biological plausibility, temporal plausibility, incorporate the major determinants of intrauterine growth and gestational duration, be based on sound empirically proven relationships, be empirically testable, incorporate direct and indirect effects, incorporate chains of risk, and plausibly explain the transformation of the social into the biological (*see* Chapter 6).
- A theoretical model of biopsychosocial pathways to birthweight at the individual level can be extended to incorporate societal level influences on risk exposure at the individual level in order to account for the observation that societies differ in their population exposure to risk factors for adverse pregnancy outcomes (*see* Chapter 7).
- The individual level model and the extended model need to be tested, modified and developed in empirical data sets; however, they provide a basis for developing new approaches to the promotion of optimal birthweight including health and social policy initiatives.

This book does not claim to offer a complete answer to the problems of promoting optimal birthweight in all populations nor is it likely that the model pathways proposed in Chapters 6 and 7 will provide the definitive framework for future successful interventions to reduce adverse pregnancy outcomes. However, it is hoped that the ideas considered in the book and the comprehensive approach combining biological and social influences on birthweight at individual and societal levels constitute a useful contribution to rethinking approaches to preventing low birthweight and preterm birth and promoting optimal population birthweight.

Addendum

Since preparing the manuscript for this book, I have become aware of a paper by Wilcox that challenges my main thesis.[1] Wilcox cites evidence to support the view that birthweight is not on the causal pathway to perinatal mortality and mean birthweight is not a useful measure of infant health at a population level. He postulates from this evidence that the association of birthweight with a range of outcomes across the life course may not be causal. He dismisses low birthweight and intra-uterine growth retardation (IUGR) as meaningful pregnancy outcomes. He acknowledges that the study of birthweight is valuable and that it may act as a marker for some other causal factor in the pathway to perinatal and subsequent health outcomes.

If Wilcox is right, measures to increase mean birthweight and to ensure that more infants are born in the optimal birthweight range may be ineffective in improving population health across the life course. He points out that optimal birthweight has a fixed relationship with mean birthweight with the result that shifting mean birthweight to the right merely shifts optimal birthweight by the same amount. Although the cut-off points used to define low birthweight ($< 2500g$) and IUGR ($< 10^{th}$ centile for gestational age) and, of course, preterm (< 37 weeks) are arbitrary divisions on the normal distribution, the existence of poor intra-uterine growth associated particularly, but not exclusively, with poor maternal nutrition is beyond dispute. The use of IUGR as a measure in chronically malnourished populations such as those in the Indian sub-continent remains valid and is akin to the use of cut-off points such as $\geqslant 2$ standard deviations below the mean to characterise population growth stunting.

At the individual level, it is difficult to see how a successful intervention to increase the birthweight of an infant will not reduce that infant's risk of adverse perinatal outcome given the close relationship of birthweight with risk. At the population level, there is evidence from a small number of studies that an increase in mean birthweight has been associated with improvements in perinatal outcome.[2,3] Contrary to Wilcox's suggestion, an increase in mean birthweight with a similar increase in the optimal birthweight may be associated with an improvement in perinatal mortality if the optimal perinatal mortality rate reduces concomitant with the shift of the optimal birthweight to the right.

In summary, given the extent and range of the association of birthweight with health outcomes across the life course as detailed in Chapters 1 and 2 of this book, it seems premature to dismiss birthweight as a causal factor in these associations. Even if not a causal agent, the remarkably close association of birthweight with life course measures of health means that it acts as a valuable and readily measured marker for other factors that lie on the causal pathway to these outcomes. The complex biopsychosocial pathways to birthweight at individual and societal levels (*see* Figure 6.11, p. 140 and Figure 7.3, p. 162) suggest that these factors may also exert their influence on health outcomes through similar complex pathways. Wilcox's suggestion of a common genetic factor is unlikely to be adequate to explain these relationships, particularly as the social gradients in birthweight and many of its determinants suggest that there are likely to be powerful environmental influences at work in the causal pathways.

Wilcox's paper represents a robust challenge to the thesis of this book. Whereas, in my view, the paper does not invalidate the book's arguments, it should provide the impetus for a critical reassessment of the role of birthweight and research projects designed to answer some of the challenging questions that it raises.

References

1 Wilcox AJ (2001) On the importance – and the unimportance – of birthweight. *International J Epidemiol.* **30**: 1233–41.

2 Elmén H, Höglund D, Karlberg P, Niklasson A and Nilsson W (1996) Birth weight for gestational age as a health indicator: birth weight and mortality measures at a local area level. *Euro J Public Health.* **6**: 137–41.

3 Bonellie SR and Rabb GM (1997) Why are babies getting heavier? Comparison of Scottish births from 1980–1992. *BMJ.* **315**: 1205.

Index